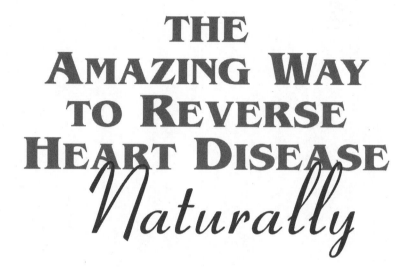

THE
AMAZING WAY
TO REVERSE
HEART DISEASE
Naturally

BEYOND THE HYPERTENSION HYPE:
WHY DRUGS ARE NOT THE ANSWER

THE
AMAZING WAY
TO REVERSE
HEART DISEASE
Naturally

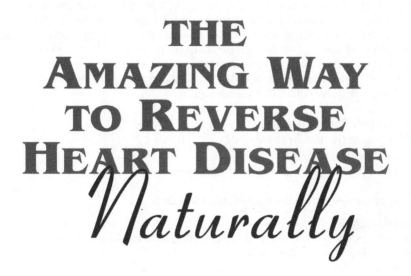

Eric R. Braverman, M.D.
with Dasha Braverman, B.S., R.P.A.-C.

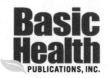

Basic Health
PUBLICATIONS, INC.

The information contained in this book is based upon the research and personal and professional experiences of the authors. It is not intended as a substitute for consulting with your physician or other healthcare provider. Any attempt to diagnose and treat an illness should be done under the direction of a healthcare professional.

The publisher does not advocate the use of any particular healthcare protocol but believes the information in this book should be available to the public. The publisher and authors are not responsible for any adverse effects or consequences resulting from the use of the suggestions, preparations, or procedures discussed in this book. Should the reader have any questions concerning the appropriateness of any procedures or preparation mentioned, the authors and the publisher strongly suggest consulting a professional healthcare advisor.

Basic Health Publications, Inc.
28812 Top of the World Drive
Laguna Beach, CA 92651
949-715-7327 • www.basichealthpub.com

Library of Congress Cataloging-in-Publication Data

Braverman, Eric R.
    The amazing way to reverse heart disease naturally / Eric R. Braverman, with Dasha Braverman.—2nd ed.
        p. cm.
    Previously published under the title: How to lower your blood pressure and reverse heart disease naturally.
    Includes bibliographical references and index.
    ISBN-13: 978-1-59120-107-6
    ISBN-10: 1-59120-107-1
    1. Heart—Diseases—Alternative treatment. 2. Heart—Diseases—Diet therapy.
    3. Dietary supplements. I. Braverman, Dasha. II. Braverman, Eric R. How to lower your blood pressure and reverse heart disease naturally. III. Title.

    RC684.A48B73   2004
    616.1'20654—dc22

                                                          2004017096

Editor: Cheryl Hirsch
Typesetting/Book design: Gary A. Rosenberg
Cover design: Mike Stromberg

Printed in the United States of America

10   9   8   7   6

Contents

Preface

This book presents a simple three-point program for reducing your blood pressure, your cholesterol, and your weight—all without drugs. The basic components of our No-More Hypertension and Heart Disease Program are:

- **The Rainbow Diet:** A nutritional plan that is low in fat, moderate in protein and nutrient-dense whole grains, and high in a cornucopia of fruits and vegetables that span the spectrum of the rainbow. Foods that are red, orange, yellow, green, blue, indigo, and violet are packed with fiber and disease-fighting antioxidants, bioflavonoids, and phytonutrients.

- **Supplement Support:** A daily supplement plan that consists of the key nutrients (fish oils, primrose oil, vitamins, minerals, and amino acids) clinically proven to slow or stop the progression of heart disease.

- **Stress Reduction, Lifestyle Changes, and Other Healing Therapies:** An essential but overlooked element that provides techniques for dealing with the primary emotional, spiritual, and lifestyle factors that contribute to heart disease, including the increased risks associated with aging.

These three components will lower the blood pressure and cholesterol, and reduce the weight of most people. Hundreds of scientific articles have appeared in mainstream medical journals from the *Journal of the American Medical Association* to the *American Medical Association News* documenting the effectiveness of this approach for treating cardiovascular disease. Following it will improve the quality of life for as many as 30 to 50 million Americans who now need one or more daily drug treatments. Even if your doctor has categorized you as "high risk," our No-More Hypertension and Heart Disease Program can return you to a normal life—you may not even need drugs—in only thirty to ninety days.

The very same program that reverses high blood pressure and elevated cholesterol also reverses heart disease. High blood pressure and elevated cholesterol are just the first steps on the way to hardening of the whole heart and cardiovascular system. The key to this program is that it will lower your blood pressure 10 to 20 points, and in most cases, will reduce your cholesterol to as low as 120. This leads to the reversal of vascular disease wherever it is in your body—from the brain to the legs to the heart. And if nutrition and supplements do not do it, then adding small changes to your lifestyle may do it, or stress-reducing exercises, or chelation treatments, and only as a last resort, drugs.

PART ONE

Understanding the Elements of Heart Disease

CHAPTER 1

The Two Precursors of Heart Disease: High Blood Pressure and Elevated Cholesterol

"**C**an there be worse sickness," asked the poet John Donne in his 1612 poem, *An Anatomy of the World,* "than to know that we are never well, nor can be so?" Donne could have been talking about heart disease, the nation's No. 1 killer, a disorder that has taken the lives of more Americans than all wars combined. It has driven patients and their doctors to despair, and to medication. Heart disease can begin as early as childhood. The truth is, you cannot start a cardiovascular health program soon enough.

"Heart disease" refers to a disorder of the heart, but in reality, it's much more than that. It implicates not just the heart, but also the 60,000-mile network of blood vessels through which the heart pushes blood with each of its 100,000 beats a day. More accurately, heart disease is a group of disorders that encompasses the heart and entire vascular system, and for this reason is often referred to as "cardiovascular disease."

Heart disease takes years to develop. For the most part, it is the result of sometimes as many as thirty years of inflammation and unseen damage to the blood vessel walls. Without any overt symptoms, artery walls can thicken and "harden" with plaque, slowly losing their flexibility. Eventually, this plaque buildup narrows the space in the arteries through which blood can flow, decreasing the supply of oxygen-carrying blood throughout the entire cardiovascular system, including the coronary arteries, which deliver blood to the heart. When hardened or narrowed, arteries are unable to supply the body's organs with what they need to function properly, which causes the heart to work harder. Another danger is that a blood clot or a piece of ruptured plaque may get stuck in an artery and deprive part of the body of its normal blood supply, causing a heart attack or stroke, the most common cardiovascular diseases. This process, called atherosclerosis, can manifest in any number of the following cardiovascular conditions:

- Myocardial infarction: This is the medical term for heart attack, the leading cause of death in the United States. Heart attack occurs when one or more of the three main coronary arteries supplying blood to the heart muscle is severely reduced or obstructed. Heart attacks usually result from atherosclerosis (also known as coronary or ischemic heart disease) and/or a blood clot lodging in a coronary artery that cuts off oxygenated blood flow to a region of the heart muscle, resulting in the death of heart tissue. Approximately 30 percent of all heart attacks are fatal.

- Stroke: The third leading cause of death in the United States. This refers to brain damage caused by a lack of blood flow to a region of the brain. Stroke is usually caused by an obstructed blood vessel due to a blood clot, which prevents oxygenated blood from getting to brain tissue, leading to the death of brain cells. Approximately 25 percent of all strokes are fatal.

- High blood pressure: The most common form of cardiovascular disease and the leading cause of stroke. Also known as hypertension, high blood pressure typically results from a loss of elasticity of the arteries. Blood pressure that is high is clinically defined as systolic blood pressure equal or greater than 140 and/or diastolic blood pressure equal or greater than 90. However, even slightly elevated blood pressure can be dangerous. Nearly two-thirds of all heart attacks occur in people whose blood pressure is only mildly elevated.

- Congestive heart failure: When a weak heart becomes unable to pump blood effectively to the rest of the body, it is called congestive heart failure, or simply heart failure. This condition can result from years of high blood pressure, atherosclerosis, a congenital heart defect (present at birth), or cardiomyopathy (a life-threatening heart condition that results from an inflammation of the muscle tissue, stiffening of the tissue, or a loss of muscle fibers).

- Peripheral vascular disease: A common complication of atherosclerosis that is caused by an insufficient supply of blood to the lower legs and feet, resulting in intense muscle pain. The peripheral vascular system consists of smaller blood vessels and capillaries in which blood clots can easily get stuck.

- Angina pectoris: Sudden pain that is typically felt in the chest or sometimes in other places like the left arm and shoulder. It is caused by impeded blood flow, leading to a shortage of oxygen to the heart tissue. The impeded blood flow is most commonly due to atherosclerosis and usually happens with exercise when the heart needs more oxygen than the body can supply.

- Intermittent claudication: This is a condition caused by poor circulation to the legs, which causes cramplike pains. It is typically the first symptom of peripheral vascular disease and can be an indication of diseased arteries elsewhere in the body.

There are many risk factors for heart disease. Genetic predisposition, advancing age, high blood pressure, diabetes, elevated LDL cholesterol and low HDL cholesterol, obesity, smoking, stress, and a sedentary lifestyle are major risk factors underlying these cardiovascular conditions. Other increasingly accepted risk factors include insulin resistance and metabolic syndrome (also known as Syndrome X), two disorders marked by elevated levels of blood sugar (glucose) and insulin, which set up a cascade of events that contribute to inflammation and plaque deposition; elevated levels of homocysteine (a potentially toxic amino acid that damages blood vessel walls); fibrinogen (a blood protein that makes platelets sticky); and C-reactive protein (a blood protein found in atherosclerotic lesions and associated with their rupture). But of all these risk factors, high blood pressure and elevated cholesterol are thought to be the two main precursors, setting the stage for the devastation to begin. Each speeds the process of atherosclerosis and its damaging life-threatening effects.

People with high blood pressure generally have high cholesterol levels. If you have hypertension, you are beginning to have heart disease. And if you have both high blood pressure and an elevated cholesterol level, you are a candidate for other serious health problems, not just to your heart and arteries, but to your kidneys, lungs, brain, and nervous system.

There is no single action you can take that will change your life as dramatically as taking control of your high blood pressure and cholesterol. Accomplish that, and you will get control of your life once more—and it's possible to do without drugs. *If you are currently on medication, do not stop without your physician's knowledge or approval.*

To learn what you can do to take charge of your cardiovascular health, you must first understand how normal blood pressure and cholesterol work, and how high blood pressure and elevated cholesterol do their damage.

UNDERSTANDING THE UPS AND DOWNS
OF BLOOD PRESSURE

Blood pressure is the pressure of the blood in the body's vascular system. The vascular system carries oxygen-rich blood away from the heart through blood vessels, arteries, and capillaries into the tissues. After the tissues are oxygenated, the blood enters the veins to be transported back to the heart and lungs. Blood pressure is a measure of the force exerted by the blood against the walls of the arteries. It is reported as a fraction. Systolic pressure, or the top number in a blood pressure reading, records the pressure caused when the heart contracts; diastolic pressure, or the lower number, indicates the pressure that occurs when the heart relaxes. Blood pressure is simply a measurement of how hard your heart has to work to circulate blood through your body.

Blood pressure is one of the two most important measurements used to assess the health of your cardiovascular system; the other is cholesterol. Read together, your systolic and diastolic numbers provide a fairly accurate picture. Blood pressure elevation (measured in millimeters of mercury, or mm Hg) is classified in stages and is more serious the higher the numbers:

BLOOD PRESSURE (mm Hg)	DESIRABLE	BORDERLINE	HYPERTENSION	
		Prehypertension	Stage 1	Stage 2
Systolic	<120	120–139	140–159	160 and above
Diastolic	<80	80–89	90–99	100 and above

High blood pressure is characterized by a reading equal or greater than 140/90. Until recently, most doctors focused on the diastolic reading (bottom number) and considered the systolic pressure (top number) only a secondary consideration in risk prevention. However, studies now show that an elevation in either one of the pressures can have dangerous implications. Incidences of stroke, heart attack, and other cardiovascular events such as aneurysm (which occurs when blood presses against a weak, thin area on a blood vessel causing it to bulge and, in some cases, to rupture) become greater at an increasing rate as systolic pressure rises. The level of systolic pressure is also important in assessing the influence of arterial pressure on cardiovascular morbidity. Males with normal diastolic pressures (<80) but elevated systolic pressures (>140) have a 2.5-fold increase in cardiovascular mortality rates when compared with individuals with normal systolic pressure (<120). Older adults with isolated high systolic pressure, a condition in which the systolic number is high even though the diastolic number is normal, and the most common form of high blood pressure in the elderly, is thought to be a significant indicator of heart attacks and strokes. As diastolic blood pressure increases from 80–89, cardiovascular events also increase. Isolated high diastolic pressure has been found to be a strong risk factor for such conditions as heart attacks and strokes, especially in younger adults.

Your blood pressure has a lot of ups and downs throughout a typical day. It can change in a matter of minutes, depending on the time of day, your psychological state, or your physical activity, for example. A reading of 120/80 when you're relaxed may rocket when you're under the pressure of visiting a doctor's office into the 140/90, above-normal, zone. This predisposition, known as "labile blood pressure" or "white coat hypertension," affects a large number of adults. Also, blood pressure may rise temporarily for a few months, as in pregnancy-induced hypertension. Only when your pressure is frequently and consistently elevated does it become true high blood pressure, or hypertension. Most people with elevated blood pressure are diagnosed with borderline blood pressure or "prehypertension." It is in this stage that the medical problems associated with high blood pressure begin, and if left untreated, can have disastrous long-term health consequences.

It's hard to believe that you could be dying if you're up and about but it's true if you have high blood pressure. That's high blood pressure–the "silent killer's"—calling card. It's painless, often symptomless, and it doesn't give you time to pack your bags. Fifty million Americans (about one out of six) have high blood pressure. This condition is even more widespread among older Americans, more than half of whom have high blood pressure. The great majority of cases presently go undetected, untreated or inadequately treated, and it's twice as life threatening if you don't know you have it. Next to old age and obesity, high blood pressure is the most potent predictor of a shortened life span. Of the 50 million Americans with high blood pressure, 10 million or more may be on medication of questionable value or that presents a documented danger.

High Blood Pressure's Effects on the Body

Chronically elevated blood pressure affects the heart and arteries the most. If your blood pressure is high it means that your heart has to work harder than normal to circulate blood through your body. Over time this adds to the wear and tear on your heart, and like any other muscle, it becomes enlarged by the extra effort, which affects its pumping action. Gradually, the heart will be less and less able to meet your body's demands and will begin to fail.

High blood pressure causes blood to circulate through your arteries at high speeds. The increased activity and strain eventually take their toll on your arteries, weakening the walls and wearing down their healthy surfaces. Lesions and patches of inflammation begin to form, which attract large amounts of harmful cholesterol, metals such as lead and cadmium, and other irritating substances, which build up over time, causing your arteries to become less elastic.

If left untreated over a period of years or decades, high blood pressure can lead to atherosclerosis, stroke, and heart failure. It can also contribute to kidney failure, diabetes, impotence, and eye conditions such as hemorrhages, retinopathy, and papilledema (swelling in the eye). Studies reported in the *Journal of the American Medical Association* (JAMA) indicate that high blood pressure can also affect brain function and is a major component of dementing diseases such as Alzheimer's and vascular dementia, the second most common form of dementia after Alzheimer's. Another complication of hypertension is that it impairs nutrient absorption from food. Because the effects of high blood pressure spread throughout the body's entire vascular system, there is ultimately no organ or system that goes untouched.

Causes of High Blood Pressure

In 90 to 95 percent of people with high blood pressure, there is no single physiological cause. This type of blood pressure is called "essential" or "primary" hypertension. Even though the precise cause of high blood pressure is not yet known, research indicates it is a complex interaction among genetic, environmental, and lifestyle-related risk factors. These primary factors are:

- Improper, poorly balanced diet, usually high in calories, sodium (salt) and fat, and low in protein and heart-protective nutrients

- Imbalanced sodium to potassium ratio

- Alcohol abuse

- Cigarette smoking

- Elevated cholesterol

- Insulin resistance

- Medications (most over-the-counter cold and flu products and prescription appetite suppressants and non-steroidal anti-inflammatory drugs)

- Obesity

- Stress

- Toxins, especially heavy metals (aluminum, cadmium, lead, and others)

Obesity is the number one lifestyle factor linked to high blood pressure, as well as to many other modern diseases. Studies have shown that increases in blood pressure are directly proportional to increases in weight. Even a loss of a few pounds has been shown to make a significant difference in reducing blood pressure.

Smoking is also another major contributing factor. Smoking just one cigarette can cause your blood pressure to climb ten points or more. Nicotine makes blood vessels constrict, which causes the heart to work harder to pump blood through the vessels, and carbon monoxide from the smoke reduces the amount of oxygen in the blood. Smoking on a regular basis can cause blood pressure to remain elevated. In time, the reduction in oxygen levels promotes the clotting of blood and the development of plaque.

A diet high in sucrose (found primarily in cane sugar and in some fruits and vegetables) also has the effect of raising blood pressure. Americans in particular consume large amounts of refined sugar. High levels of carbohydrate consumption (50 to 80 percent of the diet) have been shown to induce sodium retention and, through this retention of sodium, to raise blood pressure. Some researchers believe that the dietary factors in high blood pressure may be related to the excess intake of calories from saturated fat (found primarily in animal products), as well as high cholesterol and salt.

Stress and its activation of the sympathetic nervous system, one of two divisions of the autonomic (involuntary) nervous system, which dominates during times of stress, play an important role in creating high blood pressure. It has become increasingly clear that lifestyle changes can reduce excess levels of catecholamines, potentially harmful chemicals that increase with stress. Anxiety and emotional stress elevate blood pressure in many, but not all, individuals. And although tension is not always synonymous with hypertension, studies repeatedly show that anxiety is one emotion that causes blood pressure to jump. Your personality is also a contributing factor. The longest study of health in the United States, the legendary and ongoing Framingham Heart Study, identified that having a type-A personality (overachievers) increases your risk of high blood pressure.

Possible environmental factors associated with high blood pressure include a cold climate, differences in temperature between winter and summer, and low socio-economic status, and a low level of education. Conditions such as pregnancy at a later age (thirty-five or older) and consuming large amounts of licorice (glycyrrhizinicals) can also temporarily cause high blood pressure.

In the remaining 5 to 10 percent of cases, when high blood pressure is a symptom of an underlying disease or medical condition, it is called "secondary" hypertension. Hypertension of this type can be caused by diabetes, hypercalcemia (too much calcium in the blood), hormonal disorders (acromegaly, adrenal dysfunction, excess aldosterone production, hypo- and hyperthyroidism, Cushing's disease, estrogen use), preeclampsia (a complication of pregnancy), kidney disorders (renal artery stenosis, polycystic kidneys, interstitial kidney disease, glomerulonephritis), sleep apnea, tumors (pheochromocytoma), or coarctation of the aorta (an inherited defect of the aorta).

Who Gets High Blood Pressure

Apart from the lifestyle factors and underlying health problems that can contribute to high blood pressure, some racial groups are more likely than others to develop the condition. High blood pressure is more common in African-Americans and Hispanics than it is in Caucasians. The percentage of African-Americans with hypertension is approximately one-third higher than for whites. It is virtually an epidemic in the African-American population, where about one-third of blacks between the ages of eighteen and forty-nine and two-thirds of those over age fifty have hypertension. African-Americans still are twice as likely to suffer from kidney failure and have the world's second highest incidence of stroke, behind the Japanese.

Hypertension also affects genders differently. Men tend to develop high blood pressure earlier than women. Blood pressure in males seems to begin rising between the ages of thirty five and fifty, while in women it doesn't normally start ascending until after menopause, at which point their respective risks are similar. This rise in blood pressure during male and female menopause is associated with a decline in sex hormones, and a rise in cholesterol. The sex hormones testosterone, estrogen, and progesterone are made from cholesterol. When the body stops utilizing cholesterol to synthesize sex hormones, it naturally builds up.

Aging also puts you at greater risk. Blood pressure naturally goes up as you grow older and hypertension tends to increase with age. Blood pressure starts off at normal levels in childhood and rises gradually with age. By

> ### HEART-SMARTS: *Do You Know That . . .*
>
> ❥ The average human heart beats over 2.5 billion times in a lifetime.
>
> ❥ The average heart pumps 2,000 gallons of blood each day.
>
> ❥ The heart continues to grow in size long after you reach your full height.
>
> ❥ Emotions can influence the heart rate by triggering hormones that can affect the rate at which electrical impulses are discharged.
>
> ❥ Circulating blood delivers nutrients and oxygen to the heart, other organs, and tissues, and it helps to remove waste products, as well.
>
> ❥ More women die from heart disease than breast cancer each year.

age sixty-five, more than half of all Americans—men and women alike—have high blood pressure. While high blood pressure occurs mainly in adults, the trend with this and most of our other lifestyle-driven diseases is that children are increasingly affected as well, possibly due to dietary factors such as higher fat and refined carbohydrate consumption. And the younger you are when you get it, the more difficult the cure.

Heredity also plays a small role in hypertension. If your parents or grandparents had high blood pressure, it increases the likelihood that you will too.

UNDERSTANDING THE GOOD AND THE BAD OF CHOLESTEROL

Cholesterol is a waxy, fatlike substance that is actually necessary for your health. It is an essential component of every cell and is needed by the body to perform many basic functions. It helps the liver manufacture bile, needed for digesting fat, and is a building block from which the body makes adrenal and sex hormones. Cholesterol also forms a protective cloak around cell walls and the myelin sheaths of the nerves, and serves as a lubricant in artery walls, helping the smooth flow of blood.

The liver makes most of the cholesterol the body needs to perform these functions. If still more cholesterol is needed, it can also be derived from food sources. This type of cholesterol is known as dietary cholesterol. Once it is carried from the intestines and processed by the liver, it becomes serum, or blood, cholesterol and is combined with the cholesterol the liver makes on its own. This serum cholesterol is then distributed to cells where it is needed, throughout the body. Ideally, any extra is then returned to the liver.

Cholesterol is critical to the body in balanced amounts. Too little blood cholesterol is unhealthy, as is too much. Cholesterol levels lower than 135 can be a sign of adrenal stress, severe liver damage (due to chemicals, drugs, or hepatitis), and autoimmune or "self-attacking" disorders such as allergies, lupus, and rheumatoid arthritis. Depressed cholesterol levels have also been correlated with cancer and impaired immune function in general, which can manifest as fatigue, recurrent infections, slow wound healing, and an increased susceptibility to every type of illness. Low-fat diets and the use of street drugs or cholesterol-lowering drugs can cause cholesterol to drop to unhealthy levels, as can excessive exercise (especially in females). Psychological stress and a deficiency of essential fatty acids and the mineral manganese are other causes of abnormally low cholesterol levels.

If there is more cholesterol present than the body can process and use, cholesterol can be deposited inside the walls of blood vessels, where it becomes dangerous to the body. Elevated cholesterol, which is defined as a reading greater than 200, is the single most important risk factor in coronary heart disease. Heart disease most often involves partial or complete obstruction of one of the coronary arteries that supply the heart with oxygen. The plaque that can build up on arterial walls and result in their narrowing is composed mainly of cholesterol-rich fatty deposits, which are combined with calcium, proteins, and smooth muscle cells (fast-growing cells that proliferate on the lining of injured artery walls). This buildup triggers a cascade of events that contribute to heart disease.

The Framingham Heart Study was the first health study in the United States to find a correlation between cholesterol levels and heart disease. In this large-scale study with more than 360,000 people, findings showed that cardiovascular mortality rose steadily with increasing cholesterol levels. Besides atherosclerosis, elevated levels of cholesterol have also been implicated in gallstones, mental impairment, and high blood pressure.

The relationship between cholesterol levels and heart disease is complicated, however, by the fact that the body produces two principal forms of cholesterol. Cholesterol is carried through the bloodstream in two protein components: low-density lipoproteins (LDLs) and high-density lipoproteins (HDLs). The LDL is considered "bad," or damaging, cholesterol because it carries cholesterol from the liver to the cells of the body and blood vessels where it ends up inside cells that line the artery walls. HDL, on the other hand, is considered "good," or protective, because it transports cholesterol from the arterial walls to the liver, where it is broken down for removal from the body. LDL and HDL cholesterol also differ in their size. LDL cholesterol is made up of larger particles that are likely to get caught in an artery's lining, whereas particles of HDL cholesterol are smaller and therefore are less likely to get caught. The higher your levels of LDL cholesterol, the greater your risk of coronary heart disease.

Cholesterol's Effects on the Body

Research over the last decade is showing that cholesterol, by simply burrowing into the cells lining an artery, does not always transform into artery-clogging plaque. It is now thought that the process of oxidation is what makes the LDL component of cholesterol so harmful. Oxidation occurs when your antioxidant system cannot neutralize unstable, negatively changed molecules called free radicals. Free radicals occur naturally in the body or can be initiated by exposure to environmental pollutants such as cigarette smoke, chemicals, over-the-counter and prescription drugs, heavy metals, or stress. Without sufficient antioxidant protection, LDL cholesterol combines with oxygen to form oxy-cholesterol. This substance behaves inside the artery walls like a highly reactive free radical, where it irritates artery walls, initiates inflammation, and contributes to an eventual buildup of plaque. Left untreated, this plaque will eventually shut off the affected artery entirely or rupture and break off, leading to angina, and possibly, heart attack or stroke.

Some of the earliest studies on oxy-cholesterol were reported in the *Journal of Orthomolecular Medicine.* In experiments, rabbits were administered pure cholesterol, as well as oxy-cholesterols. After forty-five days, thickening of the lining of the aorta (the main artery conducting blood from the heart through the chest and abdomen) was observed in the oxy-cholesterol group. No thickening was observed in the rabbits that were given the pure cholesterol. The same experiment, performed on monkeys, produced similar results. Radioactively-labeled oxy-cholesterols were tracked through the body and the results showed that oxy-cholesterols were notably connected to the low-density lipoproteins (LDLs) and very low-density lipoproteins (VLDLs). VLDLs are composed mostly of triglycerides, which are even larger particles than bad LDLs. There was practically no affinity toward the good high-density lipoproteins.

Because cholesterol is a mix of good (HDL) and bad (LDL), cholesterol readings are classified according to your total cholesterol (the quantity of LDL and HDL circulating in your blood), and trigylcerides. The higher the numbers for total cholesterol, LDL cholesterol, and trigylcerides, the greater your risk of heart disease. In contrast, the higher your levels of HDL cholesterol, the lower your risk of heart problems. Readings of total blood cholesterol include both HDL and LDL levels combined and are measured in milligrams per deciliter of blood (mg/dL).

BLOOD FAT (mg/dL)	DESIRABLE (low risk)	BORDERLINE (moderate risk)	ELEVATED (high risk)
Total cholesterol	<200	200–239	240 and above
LDL cholesterol	<130	130–159	160 and above
HDL cholesterol	60 and above	35–59	<35
Trigylcerides	<200	200–399	400 and above

The best cholesterol profile is one that has a ratio of low level of LDL cholesterol to a high level of HDL cholesterol.

Causes of High Cholesterol

Blood cholesterol levels can be influenced by what you eat. If there is more cholesterol present than the body's natural mechanisms can cope with, cholesterol can be deposited on the interior walls of blood vessels, narrowing them. Because the liver uses saturated fat to manufacture cholesterol, consuming an excessive amount can significantly raise blood cholesterol levels. Fatty red meat and dairy products are primary sources of dietary cholesterol and saturated fat. In addition, saturated fats that have been left out or have been fried, smoked, cured, or aged, as well as powders of egg and moldy cheeses (found in many fast foods), contain large amounts of oxy-cholesterol and increase blood cholesterol levels. Table 4.1 on page 40 in Chapter 4 provides a list of the twelve foods highest in oxidized cholesterol. Suffice it to say that in the American diet, most harmful cholesterol intake comes from heat-damaged, oxidized fats and that most Americans eat a diet that is woefully lacking in the nutrients that can protect their arteries from the havoc caused by the oxidation of cholesterol.

The following foods and conditions contribute most to high cholesterol levels:

• Amino acid deficiency caused by poor quality protein intake

• Antioxidant deficiency (vitamins C and E, selenium, and zinc) caused by low intake of fruits and vegetables

- Deficiency in biotin and carnitine (substances related to the B vitamins) caused by processing of whole grains

- Essential fatty acid deficiency caused by poor quality fat intake

- Excess alcohol intake

- Excess hydrogenated or processed fats intake (lard, shortening, cotton-seed oil, palm oil, margarine, and others) found in many refined processed foods

- Excess starch intake (corn, white potatoes, and others)

- Excess sugar intake found in many refined processed foods

- Fiber deficiency caused by low intake of fruits and vegetables

- Food allergies

- Hormone deficiencies (testosterone, DHEA, estrogen, growth hormone, and others)

- Liver dysfunction

- Increased tissue damage due to infection, radiation, impaired liver function, or oxidative activity

Who Gets High Cholesterol

Seventy-five million Americans (nearly one out of four people) in the United States have elevated cholesterol levels—and the majority of these people don't know when they have it. Like high blood pressure, cholesterol does its damage unnoticed. For an estimated 25 percent of people who experience heart attacks, there is no warning sign.

In general, men who are older than forty-five are more prone to high cholesterol. Cholesterol levels in women are more likely to rise after age fifty-five. People who smoke, have diabetes, or a family history of premature heart disease are also at increased risk. A small group of people has a hereditary disorder known as familial hypercholesterolemia, a genetic condition characterized by abnormally high cholesterol levels.

For a minority of people high cholesterol levels do not indicate the presence of heart disease. Similarly, some people can have normal levels and yet have heart disease. Overall, however, cholesterol, like high blood pressure, is an early warning sign of impending heart and cardiovascular disease.

COPING WITH HIGH BLOOD PRESSURE
AND ELEVATED CHOLESTEROL

The good news about these bad-news disorders is that they respond well and rapidly to the right treatment. And that treatment is the drug-free No-More Hypertension and Heart Disease Program, which we have used to return over 3,000 patients to a healthy, drug-free life. It's the first safe do-it-yourself (with your doctor's consent, of course) program for lowering your blood pressure and cholesterol, without drugs, for life.

Unfortunately, this is not how most hypertension and elevated cholesterol is treated in many other practices. In mild cases of high blood pressure or slightly raised cholesterol, a regime of diet, exercise, and weight loss is sometimes advocated, but for the most part, antihypertensive medications and cholesterol-lowering drugs are almost always prescribed. And while they may be effective in bringing blood pressure and cholesterol into a healthy range, they can have unpleasant and even dangerous side effects, often sending you into a downward spiral, making you vulnerable to other heart and vascular disturbances and major organ disorders.

As you will see in the next chapter, treating your condition with these drugs is a Catch-22 situation.

CHAPTER 2

Beyond the Hypertension Hype: Why Drugs Are Not the Answer

I f you have your heart set on a long, happy, healthy, productive life—in spite of your high blood pressure and creeping cholesterol—revise your forecast if you are using drugs to reach that goal.

Reports by the American Medical Association (AMA), the American Heart Association (AHA), and the National Institutes of Health (NIH) indicate that treating your cholesterol and high blood pressure with the drugs currently in use reduces your sex drive, accelerates aging of all your major organs (heart, brain, lungs, and kidneys), and can shorten your life by more than sixteen years—particularly if you are ten or more pounds overweight, as 85 percent of all people with high blood pressure are. And that's just for starters. Here are a few other troublesome side effects caused by these drugs:

- Anxiety
- Breathing difficulty
- Constipation or diarrhea
- Depression
- Dizziness
- Fatigue
- Hair loss
- Headache

- Heart failure
- Hyperglycemia (high blood glucose)
- Indigestion
- Kidney damage
- Numbness or pain in the nerves
- Palpitations
- Sexual dysfunction
- Tinnitus (constant ringing or buzzing in the ears)

One out of every five people with high blood pressure and one out of every two people with elevated cholesterol receive conventional treatment using medication. A full 80 percent of hypertensives and 50 percent of those with high cholesterol go without any treatment at all. If you fall into any of those categories, you are one of the "walking wounded." Those who take drugs for high blood pressure are receiving treatment that masks their symptoms and, in some cases, actually raises cholesterol levels. This contributes to hardening of the arteries. In addition, when your cholesterol is high, it contributes to the inflexibility of your arteries. Rather than helping, the medications that you are taking for your elevated cholesterol may be worsening your condition. Drugs treat symptoms but do not cure disease.

THOSE BITTER PILLS:
THE HAZARDS OF PRESCRIPTION DRUGS

The following tables list the typical medications prescribed for lowering high blood pressure and cholesterol. You could be taking two, four, or more of the risky prescription drugs listed below. Don't get us wrong; it's not that all medications for high blood pressure and cholesterol are bad, in fact, drugs can be lifesaving for people who are critically ill—but vitamins and minerals are needed to counteract many of their potentially dangerous side effects. Here are the side effects you risk with each drug, and the naturally occurring substances you'll be substituting on our program to produce the same benefits without the risk.

TABLE 2.1. COMMONLY PRESCRIBED ANTIHYPERTENSIVE DRUGS
DIURETICS
• Loop diuretics: Lasix (furosemide), Demadex (torsemide), Edecrin (ethacrynic acid)
• Thiazide diuretics: Diuril (chlorothiazide), Enduron (methyclothiazide), Dyazide, Maxzide (hydrochlorothiazide/ triamterene), Hydrodiuril (hydrochlorothiazide)
• Potassium-sparing diuretics: Aldactone (spironolactone), Dyrenium (triamterene), Midamor (amiloride HCL)
• Miscellanenous diuretics: Hygroton (chlorthalidone), Lozol (indapamide)
METHOD OF ACTION: Promotes the excretion of excess water and salt through the kidneys, which lowers the amount of fluid circulating in the bloodstream, thereby easing the workload on the heart.
TYPICAL SIDE EFFECTS: Nausea; diarrhea; fatigue; dizziness or lightheadedness; muscle cramps or spasms; loss of sex drive; increased urinary excretion of potassium (except for potassium-sparing diuretics), sodium, chloride, magnesium, and calcium; decreased HDL; increased LDL cholesterol, triglycerides, and other dangerous fats; elevated uric acid and blood sugar; increased risk of arrhythmias, heart attack, and sudden death; prolonged use damages kidneys
EFFECTIVE ALTERNATIVES: Magnesium; primrose oil; safflower oil; high-protein diet

BETA-BLOCKERS, ALPHA-BLOCKERS, AND CENTRAL-ACTING AGENTS

• **Beta-blockers*:**
Inderal (propranolol), Corgard (nadolol), Lopressor/Toprol (metoprolol), Tenormin (atenolol), Zebeta (bisoprolol), and Coreg (carvedilol)

METHOD OF ACTION: Blocks adrenaline, a hormone that increases alertness, heartbeat, and blood pressure, thereby causing the heart to slow its rate and lower its output of blood, which in turn lowers blood pressure.

TYPICAL SIDE EFFECTS: Fatigue; headache; nausea; constipation; insomnia, sleep disorders; depression; impotence; bronchospasm; shortness of breath; slowed heartbeat; low blood pressure upon standing which can lead to dizziness or fainting; prolonged use increases depression and heart attack

EFFECTIVE ALTERNATIVES: CoQ_{10}; garlic; magnesium; potassium; taurine

• **Alpha-blockers:**
Cardura (doxazosin), Minipress (prazosin), Hytrin (terazosin), and others

METHOD OF ACTION: Relaxes smooth muscles in artery walls

TYPICAL SIDE EFFECTS: Dizziness; light headedness; low blood pressure upon standing which can lead to dizziness or fainting; sedation; sexual dysfunction; constipation; dry mouth; heart palpitations

EFFECTIVE ALTERNATIVES: CoQ_{10}; garlic; magnesium; potassium; taurine

• **Central-acting agents:**
Catapres (clonidine), Aldomet (methyldopa), Tenex (guanfacine), Serpasil (reserpine)

METHOD OF ACTION: Inhibits sympathetic nervous system from sending impulses that stimulate blood vessels to constrict and raise blood pressure.

TYPICAL SIDE EFFECTS: Sedation; drowsiness; sexual dysfunction; sleep disorders; nightmares; anxiety; nausea; dry mouth; muscle cramps; anemia; constipation; hypotension. Clonidine can cause hepatitis and heart failure; Reserpine can cause disabling depression.

EFFECTIVE ALTERNATIVES: CoQ_{10}; garlic; magnesium; potassium; taurine

VASODILATORS

Apresoline (hydralazine), Loniten (minoxidil), NitroQuick, Nitro-Dur (nitroglycerin), and others

METHOD OF ACTION: Dilates arteries, relaxing constricted vessels and lowering blood pressure.

TYPICAL SIDE EFFECTS: Headache; fluid retention; depression; Altered heart function such as increased heartbeat; increased risk of heart failure. Loniten can cause unwanted hair growth.

EFFECTIVE ALTERNATIVES: Calcium; garlic; magnesium; primrose oil; safflower oil; taurine; vitamin B_6

CALCIUM CHANNEL BLOCKERS

Norvasc (amlodipine), Cardizem/Dilacor/Tiazac (diltiazem), Plendil (felodipine), DynaCirc (isradipine), Adalat/Procardia (nifedipine), Cardene (nicardipine), Nimotop (nimodipine), Sular (nisoldipine), and Calan/Covera/Isoptin/Verelan (verapamil)

METHOD OF ACTION: Relaxes the blood vessels, improving blood flow.

TYPICAL SIDE EFFECTS: Headache; fatigue; dizziness; swelling of the hands, legs, or feet; slowed heartbeat; heart failure; constipation

EFFECTIVE ALTERNATIVES: Magnesium

ANGIOTENSIN-CONVERTING ENZYME (ACE) INHIBITORS

• **Angiotensin-Converting Enzyme Inhibitors:**
Lotensin (benazepril), Capoten (captopril), Vasotec (enalapril), Monopril (fosinopril), Prinivil/Zestril (lisinopril), Univasc (moexipril), Aceon (perindopril), Accupril (quinapril), Altace (ramipril), and Mavik (trandolapril)

METHOD OF ACTION: Widen arteries by interfering with the formation of angiotensin, one of the primary hormones that cause arteries to constrict.

TYPICAL SIDE EFFECTS: Fatigue; cough; nausea; impotence; rash; increased susceptibility to infection due to reduction in white blood cells; loss of protein in urine; kidney or liver damage; sodium and potassium retention; zinc and selenium depletion

EFFECTIVE ALTERNATIVES: Fish oil; primrose oil; vitamin E; zinc

• **Angiotensin II Receptor Blockers (ARBs)*:**
Atacand (candesartan), Teveten (eprosartan), Avapro (irbesartan), Cozaar (losartan), Benicar (olmesartan), Micardis (telmisartan), Diovan (valsartan)

METHOD OF ACTION: Blocks the action of angiotensin.

TYPICAL SIDE EFFECTS: Cramps; insomnia; nausea; vomiting

EFFECTIVE ALTERNATIVES: Fish oil; primrose oil; vitamin E; zinc

NEURON BLOCKERS

Ismelin (guanethidine); others

METHOD OF ACTION: Stops release of neurovascular irritants.

TYPICAL SIDE EFFECTS: Depression; severe sexual dysfunction; norepinephrine depletion at nerve ends

EFFECTIVE ALTERNATIVES: None available

TABLE 2.2. COMMONLY PRESCRIBED CHOLESTEROL DRUGS

HMG-COA REDUCTASE INHIBITORS

Lescol (fluvastatin), Lipitor (atorvastatin), Mevacor (lovastatin), Zocor (simvastatin), Pravachol (pravastatin)

METHOD OF ACTION: Blocks action of HMG-CoA, an enzyme necessary for manufacturing of cholesterol, thereby decreasing production of cholesterol in the liver.

TYPICAL SIDE EFFECTS: Abdominal pain; bloating; constipation; diarrhea; flatulence; interferes with production of CoQ_{10}; muscle pain or damage; nausea

EFFECTIVE ALTERNATIVES: Niacin, policosanol, red yeast rice extract

BILE-ACID RESINS

Colestid (colestipol), Questran (cholestyramine)

METHOD OF ACTION: Binds to cholesterol and helps it to be excreted by preventing it from being passed through the liver.

TYPICAL SIDE EFFECTS: Abdominal pain; belching; flatulence; gastrointestinal irritation and bleeding; nausea; hemorrhoidal problems

EFFECTIVE ALTERNATIVES: Niacin, guggul, policosanol, red yeast rice extract

ANTIHYPERLIPIDEMIC AGENT
Lorelco (probucol)
METHOD OF ACTION: Enhances metabolism of LDL cholesterol, lowers HDL cholesterol
TYPICAL SIDE EFFECTS: Abdominal pain; diarrhea; dizziness; heart rhythm disturbances; internal bleeding; headache; impotence; nausea
EFFECTIVE ALTERNATIVES: Fish oil

ANTILIPEMIC AGENT
Zetia (ezetimibe)
METHOD OF ACTION: Inhibits absorption of cholesterol by the small intestines.
TYPICAL SIDE EFFECTS: Back pain, arthrallgias, diarrhea, sinusitis, abdominal pain
EFFECTIVE ALTERNATIVES: Niacin, policosanol, red yeast rice extract

Diuretics

Diuretics are the most commonly prescribed drugs used to lower high blood pressure. Also known as "water pills," diuretics promote the excretion of excess fluids and salt (sodium) by interfering with the normal action of the kidneys. Increasing the output of urine reduces the amount of fluid circulating in the bloodstream, which in turn, lessens the workload on the heart because it has less volume to move around.

Despite their widespread use, diuretics have the largest variety of side effects among high blood pressure medications. As many as twenty-five documented side effects are associated with their use, including nausea, diarrhea, dizziness or lightheadedness, elevation of uric acid (which can lead to gout), loss of sexual drive, and depletion of potassium, sodium, calcium, and other minerals and electrolytes (salts found in body fluids that maintain electrical neutrality and are crucial for proper functioning of the heart). Low levels of potassium and magnesium can result in muscle cramps or spasms, fatigue, weakness, and sexual dysfunction. In addition, diuretics increase the possibility of severe life-threatening arrhythmias (irregular heart rhythms that are caused by an interference with the electrical pathways that produce the heart's rhythmic muscular contractions), and raise cholesterol, triglycerides, and other dangerous fat factors in the blood. People on diuretics have an increased risk of death due to heart attacks or sudden death (usually caused by some type of arrhythmia), and their long-term use can poison and damage the kidneys. Unfortunately, when low doses don't do the job, doctors are more likely to increase the dose rather than discontinue the medication.

There are several types of diuretics that may be prescribed for high blood pressure:

Thiazide diuretics such as Diuril (chlorothiazide), Enduron (methyclothiazide), Dyazide or Maxzide (hydrochlorothiazide, triamterene), and Hydrodiuril (hydrochlorothiaxide) are the type most commonly prescribed. Thiazide diuretic therapy can cause hypokalemia or hypomagnesemia (abnormally low levels of potassium or magnesium) in 50 percent of elderly people. Potassium and magnesium, as well as calcium, are needed to maintain a normal heart rhythm and contraction. While the problem of potassium deficiency is usually corrected, the loss of magnesium is rarely addressed.

Potassium-sparing diuretics such as Aldactone (spironolactone), Dyrenium (triamterene), and Midamor (amiloride HCL) draw water and sodium from the tissues without affecting the body's potassium balance. (Sometimes potassium-sparing diuretics can cause an excess of potassium.) Relatively mild, they are oftentimes prescribed along with a thiazide or loop diuretic (see following paragraph) to prevent the body from excreting too much potassium. These diuretics, however, increase the excretion of calcium, folic acid, and zinc.

Loop diuretics such as Lasix (furosemide), Demadex (torsemide), and Edecrin (ethacrynic acid) are a class of diuretics that work in the loop of the distal tube in your kidney. Because of their rapid action, they are more commonly used in emergency situations than for daily use.

Beta-Blockers

Beta-blockers are the second most-commonly used therapy for high blood pressure. This class of medications includes Inderal (propranolol), Corgard (nadolol), Lopressor/Toprol XL (metoprolol), Tenormin (atenolol), Zebeta (bisoprolol), and Coreg (carvedilol). Beta-blockers reduce high blood pressure by blocking nerve impulses in the beta limb of the autonomic nervous system—the part of the nervous system that governs involuntary actions. This inhibits the action of adrenaline, a hormone that increases alertness, heartbeat, and blood pressure. Adrenaline allows the heart to beat more slowly and with less force, thereby reducing its output of blood.

Beta-blockers have similar side effects to diuretics. High blood levels of undesirable lipids, impotence, and fatigue have been found in people treated with beta-blockers. Twenty-eight percent of people on Cosopt (timolol maleate), a beta-blocker used to lower blood pressure in the eye, experience adverse reactions, most commonly fatigue, dizziness, and nausea. Beta-blockers worsen asthma and increase depression. Twenty-five percent of all people on beta-blockers eventually must be treated with anti-

depressant drugs. Beta-blockers also lower levels of protective HDL cholesterol, and lipid-soluble beta-blockers such as Zebeta (bisoprolol) that cross
the blood-brain barrier (a series of semi-permeable partitions monitoring
and separating the body and its supply of substances and nutrients from
the brain) have been known to produce side effects, which are toxic to the
nervous system, and to induce cold in the extremities.

Some evidence indicates that beta-blockers are more effective for treating high blood pressure in Anglo-Americans than in African-Americans.
Nevertheless, the use of beta-blockers is not recommended for more than
two to three years at a time for most people. Used long-term, they can
weaken the heart muscle significantly and increase the risk of heart failure
or heart attack.

Alpha-Blockers

Alpha-blockers such as Minipress (prazosin), Cardura (doxazosin), and
Hytrin (terazosin) lower dopamine (a key chemical in the brain responsible
for transmitting feelings of satisfaction, arousal, and reward) and lower
blood pressure by dilating blood vessels. They may also lower total blood
cholesterol (both the "good" and "bad"), as well as triglycerides. Alpha-
blockers have a long list of side effects including dizziness, light-headedness, constipation, postural hypotension (feeling faint or actually passing
out when moving from a seated/lying to a standing position), sedation,
dry mouth, heart palpitations, and increased risk of congestive heart failure. In addition, 30 percent of all hypertensives on alpha-blockers suffer
from sexual disorders. In general, they have not been found to be particularly helpful in long-term treatment of high blood pressure.

Central-acting Agents

Central-acting agents (central adrenergic inhibitors) such as Catapres
(clonidine), Aldomet (methyldopa), Serpasil (reserpine), and Tenex (guanfacine) prevent the nervous system from sending impulses that increase
heartbeat and stimulate blood vessels to constrict. Their side effects, especially those associated with Aldomet, are more severe than the side effects
of beta-blockers or ACE inhibitors (which are discussed shortly) with regard
to drowsiness, depression, fatigue, sexual disorder, headache, neck pressure, insomnia, and nightmares. Up to 50 percent of people on one of
these three drugs experience fatigue or lethargy; up to 30 percent have
some form of sexual disorder; and over 10 percent have sleep disorder,
nightmares, headaches, anxiety, irritability, palpitations, dry mouth, dizzi-

ness, nausea, and muscle cramps. Catapres can lead to anemia, and may shorten your life span by years by inducing hepatitis and heart failure. The longer these medications are taken, the worse the side effects.

Vasodilators

As the name suggests, vasodilators cause blood vessels to dilate, thereby relaxing their walls and lowering blood pressure. These include such medications as Apresoline (hydralazine), Loniten (minoxidil), NitroQuick and Nitro-Dur (nitroglycerin), and others. The use of vasodilators is frequently accompanied by headaches. They also produce depression in 10 to 15 percent of the people taking them. Other side effects of vasodilators are fluid retention, heart-rhythm problems, and an increased risk of coronary heart disease. Loniten can cause unwanted hair growth and Apresoline can deplete the mineral manganese from the body. Manganese is necessary for fat metabolism, a healthy immune system, and blood sugar (glucose) regulation. A deficiency of this mineral boosts blood pressure, and may lead to atherosclerosis and seizures. Vasodilators are frequently prescribed with a diuretic and beta-blocker.

Calcium Channel Blockers

Included in this group are drugs such as Norvasc (amlodipine), Cardizem, Dilacor, Tiazac (diltiazem), Plendil (felodipine), DynaCirc (isradipine), Cardene (nicardipine), Nimotop (nimodipine), Sular (nisoldipine), Calan, Covera, Isoptin, Verelan (verapamil), and Adalat and Procardia (nifedipine). Also called calcium antagonists, calcium channel blockers ease the heart's workload by slowing down the passage of nerve impulses—and hence the contractions—of the heart muscle, and by blocking the transfer of calcium into smooth-muscle cells. Smooth muscle cells are cells that begin to grow on the lining of artery walls damaged or injured by free radicals. If allowed to grow, they will eventually choke off blood flow. These medications improve blood flow through the heart and throughout the cardiovascular system, reduce blood pressure, correct irregular heartbeat, and help prevent angina pain.

Calcium channel blockers, when compared to diuretics and/or beta-blockers, are considered to be more efficient and to result in fewer side effects. However, they too can cause a range of side effects, including swollen ankles, constipation, fatigue, headache, and dizziness. On the down side of calcium channel blockers, several studies have associated them with higher rates of acute heart attacks and heart failure.

ACE Inhibitors

Angiotensin-converting enzyme (ACE) inhibitors inhibit production of angiotensin, a hormone that is a potent blood-vessel constrictor, thus relaxing the vessels and lowering blood pressure. Members from this class of drugs include Lotensin (benazepril), Capoten (captopril), Vasotec (enalapril), Monopril (fosinopril), Prinivil, Zestril (lisinopril), Univasc (moexipril), Aceon (perindopril), Accupril (quinapril), Altace (ramipril), and Mavik (trandolapril).

The newest class of ACE inhibitors is known as angiotensin II receptor blockers or ARBs. Examples of these medications include Diovan (valsartan), Atacand (candesartan), Teveten (eprosartan), Avapro (irbesartan), Cozaar (losartan), Benicar (olmesartan), and Micardis (telmisartan). ARBs work to lower blood pressure by blocking the action of angiotensin rather than by preventing its formation. This blocking action stops the angiotensin from tightening the arteries and raising blood pressure.

Possible side effects of both ACE inhibitors and ARBs include fatigue, decreased sexual desire or impotence, cough, potassium retention, rash, and reduced reserves of copper, zinc, selenium, and other trace minerals that help protect your immune system. Ace inhibitors are not recommended for people with severe liver or kidney disease. However, in general, side effects tend to be less of a problem with ACE inhibitors than with other antihypertension drugs, especially because they do not promote insulin resistance, a condition in which the body does not respond to insulin properly. In diabetics for whom this is a serious problem, ACE inhibitors actually protect the kidneys.

Cholesterol-lowering Medications

HMG-CoA reductase inhibitors, also known as statin drugs, are the most popular of the cholesterol-lowering medications. Examples include Lescol (fluvastatin), Lipitor (atorvastatin), Mevacor (lovastatin), Pravachol (pravastatin), and Zocor (simvastatin). These drugs work by slowing down the activity of HMG-CoA, an enzyme that is needed to manufacture cholesterol in the liver.

Cholesterol-lowering medications are costly, and in some people can cause serious problems such as muscle disease or muscle breakdown. Because these drugs work in the liver, people using them must have their blood tested routinely to monitor liver function. Other potential side effects include abdominal pain, bloating, constipation, diarrhea, flatulence, muscle pain, and nausea. They also interfere with production of coenzyme Q_{10}, one of the most important nutrients for proper functioning of the heart muscle.

Cholesterol-lowering drugs are associated with increased accidents, because of depletion of serotonin (a mood-elevating neurotransmitter that also has relaxing and sedative properties). So, while the drugs may lower your cholesterol, you pay a price in the brain. The objective is this: when heart disease is treated with these drugs, be sure to build up the brain simultaneously, thus avoiding the deleterious effects of the drugs on the nervous system. Previously, some cholesterol-lowering drugs have been linked to increased cancer and overall health problems. A lowered blood pressure is obtained when cholesterol is lowered, but this should be done naturally, or with careful attention to maintaining healthy brain chemistry.

A whole array of new symptoms and side effects manifest themselves with the use of standard pharmacological medications for high blood pressure and elevated cholesterol. As you've seen, most drugs for high blood pressure kill your sex drive, interfere with normal brain function, decrease alertness and memory, cause depression, deplete the body's stores of the essential heart minerals potassium and magnesium, elevate cholesterol, triglycerides, and other dangerous fats, and damage the circulatory system in the long run. Even the best of the high-blood pressure drugs, the so-called angiotensin-II receptor blockers, worsen the quality of life for 30 to 40 percent of all people. And if you are elderly, you are especially vulnerable to detrimental effects on cerebral functioning. Approximately 30 to 50 percent of elderly people experience side effects from high blood pressure-drug therapy. Rapid treatment of high blood pressure in the elderly can cause quick drops in blood pressure and possibly lead to stroke. Antihypertensive drugs in the elderly have also been associated with the genesis of acute as well as chronic pancreatitis (inflammation of the pancreas). According to a recent report in the *Journal of the American Medical Association,* lifestyle changes and low-dose diuretics should be the first choice in treatment of high blood pressure in the elderly.

The great many side effects of medications for the treatment of high blood pressure and/or elevated cholesterol, as well as the financial strain of a lifetime of prescription drug use, cause many cases of noncompliance with the regimen and ineffective long-term therapy, doctors find. For the great majority of people, the side effects may far outweigh the potential gain.

A DAY IN THE LIFE OF A HYPERTENSIVE WITH ELEVATED CHOLESTEROL

Drugs are a large part of the day for many of the nation's 50 million victims of the country's most devastating but least understood threat. Are you one of them? If you are, how familiar does the following scenario sound?

7 A.M.: Time to get up and take your first blood pressure reading of the day. It's 150/90, ten points lower than last night and still in the "mild" range. So far, so good. Now for breakfast—first "deprivation" meal of the day. Because salt, fat, cholesterol, and extra calories are all risk factors, according to your doctor, breakfast consists of a glass of fruit juice, one thin slice of unbuttered whole-wheat toast, scrambled eggs (whites only) seasoned with a salt substitute, and a cup of decaffeinated coffee with a nonfat, nondairy creamer. To reduce the volume of fluids in your body and remove excess sodium, you take your first diuretic of the day, and prepare for one of the several side effects you usually experience.

What will it be today? The overwhelming lethargy that puts you to sleep on your hour's commute to the office? Will you feel washed out all day? Will you experience the rippling muscle spasms in your legs and feet that sometimes paralyze you—right in the middle of an important meeting with a new client or the boss? Or will it be a further reduction in sexual stamina—ruining something that used to be the high point of your hard-working day?

Next, some mild, doctor-prescribed, midmorning exercise—perhaps a brisk walk or slow bicycle ride to a nearby city park and back or low-impact aerobics—to help regulate your heart rhythm. Intense exercise, which boosts blood pressure to 200/100 and accelerates heartbeat, can be dangerous. A gradual elevation in blood pressure is more desirable. You hope as you exercise you won't experience any dizziness, one of the side effects caused by the HMG-CoA reductase inhibitor you're taking.

12:00 P.M.: You get ready for your second meal and second drug of the day. Today your lunch is canned no-sodium cream of celery soup with salt-free crackers and a piece of fresh fruit to supply the fiber and minerals which, according to your doctor, you lack when you're hypertensive. You open a salt-free seltzer to down drug number two—a beta-blocking agent. You remind yourself why you need this pill; according to the doctor, it's the only way to prevent a buildup of excess adrenaline, which boosts blood pressure. Yet the beta-blocker often makes you depressed, sometimes nauseous or dizzy. You hope that today it only makes you a little groggy.

Finishing your seltzer, you remember that your doctor has added a second drug you must take with your midday meal—a vasodilator, which serves the purpose of opening up and relaxing constricted arteries and blood vessels. And because a vasodilator can cause rapid and extreme water retention, there's another diuretic to take. It's hard to know what's worse—the water retention itself or the drug that counteracts it.

7:00 P.M.: Dinner won't exactly make your day either, especially since you like to eat. After a no-cocktail hour (alcohol and caffeine—both blood pressure boosters—are off the menu) you sit down to a dinner you might have enjoyed if you weren't on medication: filet of flounder, broiled and served with a no-fat wine sauce, a baked potato and steamed green beans—plus a 95 percent fat-free, imitation ice cream. But the prospect of downing another drug—this time an ACE inhibitor—takes the pleasure out of the meal. Side effects may stop at a dry mouth if you're lucky, but you've read the medical literature and this one's a bitter pill to swallow. According to the *Physician's Desk Reference,* side effects of ACE inhibitors include possible kidney failure, loss of protein in the urine, and increased risk of heart attack and a shortened life span. Most common side effects are fatigue and sexual dysfunction, and these are the least severe. It takes more than a little bit of sugar to make medicine like this go down, especially if you are not taking your vitamins to counteract many of the side effects.

10:00 P.M.: And bedtime isn't the happy prospect it used to be either, since the last thing you will be enjoying is sex or a good read—thanks to the pre-lights out medication your doctor just added to the menu. This one, a central-acting agent, lowers blood pressure by changing the way your sympathetic nervous system works. Unfortunately, you've discovered it also reduces sexual drive and performance, just like the diuretics you take.

Your wife says she understands that your temporary impotence is a side effect of these drugs—but does she? And do you really need all these drugs? You ask yourself this every day. How much damage are they doing to the rest of your body, you wonder? And how long will you be taking them?

A day like the one described above—one that millions of men and women face every day—is better than dying. But there are more pleasurable ways to spend the next twenty-four hours—and the rest—of your life, even if you have high blood pressure and elevated cholesterol.

BUT THAT'S NOT ALL

Taking one drug almost inevitably leads to the taking of another. If an individual drug fails to bring your blood pressure and/or cholesterol under control, then two or more different medications are usually combined to achieve a greater effect. This is called the "stepped care" approach to high blood pressure and heart disease.

In this typical scenario, a drug is prescribed, usually a diuretic and, if needed, a cholesterol-blocking agent, along with some general dietary information to help reduce salt intake and weight, if needed. After one month or so, if treatment doesn't work, your doctor will either prescribe a bigger dose or an additional drug such as a beta-blocker or a calcium channel blocker. If, after another month or so, these drugs fail to bring blood pressure and cholesterol under control, your doctor will add another drug, probably an ACE inhibitor or angiotensin receptor blocker (ARB), and a more powerful cholesterol drug known as an antilipemic, which will require juggling the doses of the other drugs you're taking. It's a vicious circle. Once drug regimens are opted for, drug therapies will spiral. Depending on your condition and your physician, you may be taking as few as one or as many as a dozen medications a day.

To make matters even worse, statistics on traditional drug therapies for hypertension and high cholesterol show they are not solving the problem. Here are a few of the sad facts:

- More than $28 billion is spent annually on prescriptions for heart and blood pressure drugs, the largest medical expenditure for a disease condition in the United States. Among these, statins account for almost $14 billion worth of sales.

- Twenty-six percent of people using antihypertensives continue to have high blood pressure.

- Out of 14 percent of the people using cholesterol drugs to treat their elevated cholesterol, only 7 percent bring their cholesterol levels within the recommended limits.

- Only a certain small percentage of formerly treated hypertensives maintain normal blood pressure when treatment is stopped. After abrupt withdrawal from antihypertensive medications, blood pressure usually rebounds and the need for drugs continues to increase.

- Despite medical advances in diagnosis and treatment, deaths resulting from high blood pressure have increased in the past decade.

This is why a more effective approach to high blood pressure and heart disease is necessary. Ironically, the *Annals of Internal Medicine* and the *American Medical Association News* have finally suggested that dietary and lifestyle changes, *not* drugs, are the best option and that the focus of treatment for high blood pressure and elevated cholesterol should move toward the elimination of pharmacological drugs to reduce the risk factors for heart disease. According to an article in the *Journal of the American Medical Association*, "Nutritional therapy may substitute for drugs in a sizeable group of people with high blood pressure, and if drugs are still needed, it can lessen some unwanted biochemical effects of drug treatment." One study in Finland found that death from heart disease was cut by 49 percent in some segments of the population simply by restructuring the diet. Nutrition and lifestyle have now entered into orthodox medical thinking as viable options for the treatment of high blood pressure and heart disease.

Instead of the traditional, stepped-care approach, your first step should be to address the nutritional, biochemical, and environmental causes of your high blood pressure and heart disease.

CHAPTER 3

What's the Alternative?

You can't afford to take the wrong steps or to take no steps at all. Even the slightest elevation in blood pressure and cholesterol cannot be dismissed and studies indicate that blood pressure that yo-yos may be more dangerous than blood pressure that remains consistently high.

Do you want to keep footing the bill for a lifetime of medicine that, ironically enough, increases your risk of heart attack, stroke, and early death? Such "help" doesn't come cheap. The cost of controlling high blood pressure and cholesterol with medication can run into hundreds of thousands of dollars over a lifetime. And that expense can climb even higher if the cost of treating the side effects produced by such drugs is considered, as well.

If you're sick of being sick and are ready to consider a cost-sensible alternative with a near 100 percent return in terms of health benefits and financial relief, you're ready to try the No-More Hypertension and Heart Disease Program.

The No-More Hypertension and Heart Disease Program gets results whether you are suffering from mild, borderline, or even severely high blood pressure. It has been shown to lower blood pressure as high as 180/120 to 120/80, total cholesterol as high as 400 to 180, and triglycerides as high as 1,000 to 200 or less—in thirty-to-ninety days. People seventy-five or older may experience less dramatic results due to a more advanced stage of the disease.

Even if your doctor has categorized you as "high risk," our program can return you to a normal life—in only thirty to ninety days.

Here's how:

• By replacing high-risk foods that make cholesterol and high-blood pressure with no-risk foods that break cholesterol- and high-blood pressure, using the Rainbow Diet.

- By replacing dangerous cholesterol and high blood pressure-lowering drugs with safe cholesterol and high-blood pressure-lowering supplements that work like drugs—but without the health-damaging side effects.

- By breaking the bad habits that set you up for heart disease and high blood pressure in the first place (smoking, overeating, stress, inactivity, and too much salt, sugar, alcohol, and caffeine), and starting on a daily stress control and easy exercise plan.

Ninety-five percent of patients on our treatment program have succeeded in becoming drug-free within a few weeks. You can, too. If your condition is severe, you may need to continue your medication temporarily. It is important that you never change or stop taking your medication without your physician's knowledge or approval. Monitor your progress in partnership with your doctor, who will advise you when your medications are no longer needed.

If you need drugs temporarily, work with your physician to determine whether the drugs you're on are the best for you. Consider using magnesium in conjunction with a calcium channel-blocker such as Procardia, Cardizem, or Calan, which is probably the best medicine for hypertension, and can be even more effective when combined with a total health program. Virtually any case of high blood pressure, high cholesterol, or obesity can be helped—and usually solved—with this program. Yours can, too, if you continue to work at it.

What sets our program apart from most other heart disease and blood pressure control programs is that it utilizes foods, supplements, and lifestyle changes to return you to health rather than one single magic key like the "right" food or a "miracle vitamin". The result is the restoration of biochemical balance to the whole body—not just to the health of your vascular system—because in high blood pressure and heart disease, the mechanisms involved in these conditions can be multiple and can affect many organs.

The No-More Hypertension and Heart Disease Program helps to restore normal functioning to the following key organs and body systems in these ways:

- Heart: Prevents free-radical damage to heart muscle; improves blood flow to the heart; helps the heart's pumping action; and strengthens and steadies the heartbeat.

- Arteries and peripheral blood vessels: Improves circulation; strengthens blood vessel walls; reduces circulating blood volume; makes blood platelets less sticky and less likely to form clots in the bloodstream; dilates arteries and improves their flexibility; protects arteries against inflammation and free-radical damage; lowers levels of harmful LDL cholesterol, triglycerides, homocysteine, and fibrinogen; increases protective HDL cholesterol; and promotes the excretion of toxic chemicals and heavy metals.

- Kidneys: Increases blood flow to the kidneys; reduces retention of sodium; and decreases fluid retention

- Liver: Improves ability to metabolize and eliminates cholesterol and other toxic waste.

- Pancreas: Helps to stabilize blood sugar by slowing the absorption of carbohydrates; regulates insulin production; decreases production of cholesterol, triglycerides, free radicals, and inflammatory chemicals; prevents storage of excessive sugar as fat.

- Thyroid: Balances fluctuations in blood pressure caused by the overproduction or underproduction of the thyroid hormone thyroxin; helps the pancreas to maintain stable blood sugar and improve insulin response; helps to control the rate at which calories and energy are expended.

- Adrenals: Rejuvenates exhausted adrenal glands overused from prolonged or recurrent stress; increases production of DHEA (dehydroepiandrosterone), which serves as the precursor for many adrenal hormones, including the stress hormone cortisol, and the sex hormones estrogen, progesterone, and testosterone; and improves physical and psychological well-being.

- Ovaries and testes: Builds up estrogen, progesterone, and testosterone to healthy levels; improves circulation; and enhances sex drive and performance.

- Brain: Helps to regulate the autonomic and sympathetic nervous systems; increases production of neurotransmitters that regulate mood, emotions, sleep, and cravings for sweets and refined carbohydrate foods; and promotes brain-wave activity associated with relaxation.

The No-More Hypertension and Heart Disease program will work no matter how much your story differs from the successful case histories you will read about in Chapter 9. Owing to the fact that no two victims of high blood pressure and/or elevated cholesterol are alike, sex, heredity, age, and lifestyle factors are all variables to be considered as you customize the program to meet your needs.

Here's what you can expect to gain from trying the No-More Hypertension and Heart Disease Program:

- Improved blood pressure

- Improved cholesterol levels

- A stronger heart

- Balanced weight loss

- Balanced blood sugar

- Elimination of toxic heavy metals

- Improved immune response

- Increased lifespan

- Increased sexual desire and performance

- Greater sense of well-being

- Reduced stress and anxiety

- Greater desire to exercise

- Balanced weight gain

- Relief from hidden food allergies (a blood pressure booster)

- Better understanding of high-quality supplements

- Learning the latest research in nutrition

- Learning healthy and delicious recipes

The No-More Hypertension and Heart Disease Program is proof that every day can be worth living, even with high blood pressure or heart disease. The Rainbow Diet, vitamin and mineral supplements, stress reduction strategies, and simple lifestyle changes will give you a feeling of well-being that supercedes how you felt before you became ill. You will be surprised at how good you can feel. You will learn: how to eat the right way with appetizing menus; how "healthy" fats can replace diuretics and beta-blockers; how the mineral niacin can replace vasodilators; how supplements in general can replace drugs safely and effectively; and, if needed, how chelation and hormone therapies can revitalize your arteries, tired glands, and the rest of your body.

No *one* factor alone can alter your already adversely altered body chemistry—but the right combination can. If you care enough to follow our simple step-by-step advice in the upcoming chapters, you can turn your health around in one to three months' time.

PART TWO

The No-More Hypertension and Heart Disease Program

CHAPTER 4

The Rainbow Diet: How It Works

O ne of the best nutritional approaches to controlling high blood pressure and heart disease is the Rainbow Diet™. It is an eating plan that is based on incorporating the seven major colors of the rainbow—red, orange, yellow, green, blue, indigo and violet—into the foods you eat. Fruits and vegetables of all colors are packed with disease-fighting nutrients. No blend of supplements can equal the benefits you can get from eating these fresh foods. Visualize a rainbow of fruits and vegetables, add lean protein (especially fish), fiber-rich whole grains, legumes (beans), healthy fats and oils, and lots of spices and herbs, and you're home free. These natural bounties are the essential ingredients of the Rainbow Diet. In this chapter, we will teach you how to use these nutrient-rich whole foods to achieve your optimal weight, and to improve your blood pressure, cholesterol, and your overall cardiovascular health.

Following are some of the highlights of the Rainbow Diet:

- Very high in vegetables

- High in fruits

- Moderate in fiber-rich whole grains

- Moderate in protein

- Low in saturated fat and cholesterol

- Low in sodium (salt)

- Low in refined grains

- Low in non-healthful oils

- Low in sugar-rich foods and beverages

- Absent in refined grains

- Absent in hydrogenated oils and trans fat

The basic principles of the Rainbow Diet are founded on a growing body of evidence from a number of large studies in Europe and the United States showing that diets consisting of whole grains, fruits and vegetables, and healthy fats and oils prevent the development of high blood pressure and heart disease. Cultures throughout the world with a tradition of eating this way—Asia, and the Mediterranean regions of Italy, Greece, and Spain—have low rates of hypertension and heart disease, and enjoy longer, healthier lives. Here in the United States, where people consume large amounts of meat and dairy products (high in cholesterol and saturated fats) and excessive amounts of processed foods (high in refined-grain carbohydrates, sugar, salt, and hydrogenated fats and oils), there is an extremely high rate of high blood pressure and heart disease. Sadly, the standard American diet is one of the biggest enemies of a healthy heart and cardiovascular system.

The Rainbow Diet is an eating plan that promotes healthy food choices that will stick with you for life. Just as eating too much of the wrong kinds of proteins, carbohydrates, and fats can lead to hypertension and heart disease, eating the right kinds of foods from these basic nutrient groups can slow, stop, or even reverse these conditions. The Rainbow Diet emphasizes learning how to discriminate between healthy and unhealthy sources of protein, carbohydrates, and fats, and learning how to eat these foods in sensible, healthy proportions.

You can use the image of a rainbow to guide you toward colorful, healthful foods and away from those foods without any color in them that are enemies of the heart and cardiovascular system. A rainbow contains red, orange, yellow, green, blue, indigo, violet, but no white! Avoid all "white foods." White foods are foods like white flour, bread, butter, salt, sugar, white rice, white pasta, and margarine—highly refined, processed foods that have been stripped of fiber and nutrients. These types of food are the main source of carbohydrates in the American diet.

White foods are generally poor choices for fulfilling your daily carbohydrate intake. Not only are these foods mostly empty calories that promote weight gain and are of no redeeming nutritional value, they are also relatively high on the glycemic index. A food's glycemic index measures the rate at which it breaks down into sugar (glucose) in the bloodstream. Eating too many high-glycemic foods causes blood sugar levels to soar, and in response to this jump in blood sugar, the hormone called insulin spikes in order to bring your blood sugar down to a healthy level. Insulin delivers blood sugar to the cells to use as fuel. While these "bad" carbohydrates provide you with quick energy, if your cells are subjected to frequent over-doses of sugar and refined-grain (or simple) carbohydrates, eventually they lose their ability to respond appropriately to insulin. When this happens, the pancreas continues to oversecrete insulin and its levels remain constantly high. Elevated insulin is known to raise cholesterol and triglyceride levels; it promotes the retention of sodium, aggravates the sympathetic nervous system, and generates a lot of free radicals and inflammatory chemicals. Any excess blood sugar not absorbed by the cells is converted into body fat. All of these are factors that increase blood pressure and your risk of heart disease and diabetes. In contrast, "good" carbohydrates are typically whole-grain (or complex) carbohydrates with a moderate or low-glycemic index. These carbohydrates have a slow, low, and steady effect on blood sugar and insulin levels and come from mainly whole grains, vegetables, and many fruits.

The Rainbow Diet emphasizes whole foods—100 percent pure, un-processed food—containing no additives, preservatives, artificial ingredients, or harmful substances. Approximately 80 percent of a typical day's menu on the Rainbow Diet consists of plant-based complex carbohydrates and 20 percent protein and fat, or amino-acid based, foods. In contrast, the daily intake of the typical American diet contains only 22 percent complex carbohydrates, and a whopping 42 percent protein and fat. By following these rainbow guidelines, you will naturally eliminate the types of foods from your diet that have been found to do the most to create high blood pressure and heart disease (as well as all other degenerative diseases) and you will consume more of those foods found to most effectively reverse these conditions. Table 4.1 on page 40 lists the top dozen offenders.

Before providing you with a two-week menu plan and some recipes to get you started, we'd like to explain the rationale for the types of foods used in the Rainbow Diet and why they are so beneficial for lowering your blood pressure, your cholesterol, and your risk of heart disease.

RAINBOW BASICS

The good news about the Rainbow Diet is that you don't have to count calories, tally fat grams, or weigh your food. There are no complicated food exchange charts to follow. If you are overweight, you will lose weight naturally on this diet as your system resumes its normal functioning and recovers its balance in response to the therapeutic doses of nutrients and special foods.

For easy reference, Table 4.5 on page 62 provides a quick guide to the

| TABLE 4.1. THE TOP 12 HYPERTENSION- AND CHOLESTEROL-MAKING FOODS ||
HYPERTENSION-MAKING FOOD	OXY-CHOLESTEROL-MAKING FOODS
Alcohol	Bacon
Caffeine	Brains
Cakes and pastries	Butter
Canned foods	Cheese (grated)
Cheese	Egg products
Pickled foods	Fast foods containing butter and eggs
Pork	Lard
Red meat	Milk powder
Salted foods	Parmesan cheese
Smoked foods	Pork chops
Sugar	Radiated food (gamma-radiation)
White flour	Salami

types of foods included and excluded on the Rainbow Diet and the number of times a day to eat from each food group. For the average person with high blood pressure who has elevated cholesterol and excess weight this breaks down to eating protein, approximately two to three times a day; good fats, one to two times a day; healthy carbohydrates in the form of fruits, two to three times a day; vegetables, four to six times a day; and grains, one to two times a day. Be moderate and use common sense in determining the size of your portions.

Since plant-based foods (fruits, vegetables, whole grains, beans and legumes) are the foundation of the diet, let's begin with them.

Fruits and Vegetables

Fruits and vegetables are the foundation of the Rainbow Diet, and for good reason. Not only are these whole foods rich in nutrients such as magnesium, potassium, and fiber, they are also naturally low in calories, fat, and sodium, and are free of cholesterol. The average American eats about three servings of fruits and vegetables a day.

Although no food or food combination has yet been clinically proven to prevent or retard disease in people, research strongly suggests that in contrast to diets high in meat, a diet rich in fruits and vegetables can help prevent and control high blood pressure and elevated cholesterol, thereby protecting against the risk of heart disease.

One well-known study involving more than 100,000 men and women from the Nurses' Health Study and the Health Professionals Follow-Up Study found that, compared to those who consumed the least number of fruits and vegetables a day, those who consumed the most had a 30 percent lower risk of ischemic stroke (the most common kind of stroke caused by a blood clot in an artery leading to the brain). In this study, the greatest protection seemed to be derived from eating citrus fruits, leafy green vegetables, and cruciferous vegetables, of which broccoli, cabbage, cauliflower, and Brussels sprouts were the most beneficial.

In another well-known study called the Dietary Approaches to Stop Hypertension (DASH) study, people with high blood pressure were divided into groups. One group ate a typical American diet, which derived 40 percent of its calories from fat and contained three servings of fruits and vegetables a day, while the other group also ate a diet that was much lower in fat and nearly three times higher in fruits and vegetables. High blood pressure dropped significantly in the group consuming the greater quantity of produce, but not at all in the group eating foods typical of the American diet. The findings showed that the higher the blood pressure, the greater the drop.

The disease-preventing effect of fruits and vegetables has been attributed to their naturally high antioxidant content (specific vitamins, minerals, and enzymes that protect cells against free radical damage) and phytochemicals (biologically active substances in plants that are responsible for giving them color, flavor, and disease-fighting power). Fruits and vegetables are also high in potassium, which is essential for keeping blood pressure in a healthy range, as well as fiber and pectin (a form of dietary fiber). Fiber and pectin bind with substances that generally result in the manufacture of cholesterol, and rid the body of these substances. They are also good for lowering LDL cholesterol, stabilizing blood sugar levels, and removing unwanted metals and toxins from the body.

Table 4.2 on page 42 highlights the specific health-promoting nutrients of fruits, vegetables, and other plant-based foods.

All fruits and vegetables have health benefits. The Rainbow Diet emphasizes a slightly higher intake of vegetables than fruits. This is because most fruits are simple carbohydrates, as well as high-glycemic foods, and they break down into blood sugar more quickly causing the release of insulin. In choosing which fruits and vegetables to eat, variety is the key. Pears, apples, bananas, and grapefruit are the best low-glycemic fruits. But it's more important to include a wide range of fruits from the entire fruit family, including apricots, peaches, plums, berries (blueberries, blackberries,

TABLE 4.2. HEALTH-PROMOTING PROPERTIES IN FRUITS, VEGETABLES, AND OTHER PLANT-BASED FOODS

Component: Allylic sulfides

Disease-fighting Properties: Lowers blood pressure by dilating blood vessels; inhibits platelet aggregation; lowers cholesterol by reducing total cholesterol and LDL cholesterol, and raising HDL cholesterol; prevents atherosclerosis by preventing oxidative reactions; promotes production of nitric oxide; protects against carcinogens by stimulating production of detoxification enzymes in the cells lining the arteries; has antibiotic and antiviral properties

Food Sources: Garlic and onions

Component: Anthocyanidins

Disease-fighting Properties: Acts as strong antioxidant; reduces LDL cholesterol; strengthens blood vessels; thins blood, boosts immune activity

Food Sources: Grapes

Component: Carotenoids

Disease-fighting Properties: Has strong antioxidant properties and cell differentiation agents (cancer cells are nondifferentiated)

Food Sources: Apricots, cantaloupe, carrots, citrus fruits, parsley, sweet potatoes, spinach, kale, turnip greens, winter squash, yams

Component: Catechins

Disease-fighting Properties: Has antioxidant properties linked to lower rates of gastrointestinal cancer (mechanisms not understood)

Food Sources: Berries, green tea

Component: Fiber

Disease-fighting Properties: Lowers cholesterol by binding with substances that manufacture cholesterol, and ridding these substances from the body; stabilizes blood sugar levels; removes toxic metals from the body; dilutes carcinogenic compounds in colon and speeds them through digestive system, thus discouraging growth of harmful bacteria while bolstering healthful ones

Food Sources: Whole grain cereals and flours, brown rice, agar-agar, all kinds of bran, most fresh fruits and vegetables, dried prunes, nuts, popcorn, seeds (especially flaxseed), beans, lentils, and peas

Component: Flavonoids

Disease-fighting Properties: Blocks receptor sites for certain hormones that promote cancers

Food Sources: Most fruits and vegetables, including parsley, carrots, citrus fruits, broccoli, cabbage, cucumbers, squash, yams, tomatoes, eggplants, peppers, soy products, berries

Component: Genistein

Disease-fighting Properties: Reduces cholesterol; acts as antioxidant; blocks growth of new blood vessels essential for some tumors to grow and spread; deters proliferation of cancer cells; eases menopausal problems

Food Sources: Soybeans, soy flour, soymilk, tofu, textured soy protein, and to a lesser extent, Brussels sprouts, cabbage, and cauliflower

Component: Indoles

Disease-fighting Properties: Acts as antioxidant; induces protective enzymes; excretes toxins, increases immune activity

Food Sources: Broccoli, Brussels sprouts, cabbage, cauliflower, and their relatives

Component: Isothiocyanates

Disease-fighting Properties: Induces protective enzymes

Food Sources: Mustard, horseradish, radishes

Component: Limonoids

Disease-fighting Properties: Induces protective enzymes

Food Sources: Citrus fruits

Component: Linolenic acid

Disease-fighting Properties: Regulates prostaglandin production

Food Sources: Many leafy vegetables and seeds, especially flaxseed

Component: Lycopene

Disease-fighting Properties: Has antioxidant properties; may aid in metabolism of cholesterol; improves enlarged prostate

Food Sources: Tomatoes, red grapefruit, watermelon

Component: Magnesium

Disease-fighting Properties: Regulates heartbeat; dilates blood vessels; prevents excess calcium from building up in arteries; promotes smooth transmission of nerve and muscle impulses

Food Sources: Almonds, apples, apricots, bananas, brown rice, garlic, leafy green vegetables, soybeans, whole grains

Component: Monoterpenes

Disease-fighting Properties: Has some antioxidant properties; inhibits cholesterol production in tumors; aids protective enzyme activity

Food Sources: Parsley, carrots, broccoli, cabbage, cucumbers, squash, yams, tomatoes, eggplant, peppers, mint, basil, citrus fruits

Component: Pectin

Disease-fighting Properties: Lowers LDL cholesterol; removes unwanted metals and toxins from the body

Food Sources: Apples, bananas, beets, cabbage, carrots, citrus fruits, and okra

Component: Phenolic acids (tannins)

Disease-fighting Properties: Has some antioxidant properties; inhibits formation of nitrosamine (a carcinogen); affects enzyme activity

Food Sources: Parsley, carrots, broccoli, cabbage, tomatoes, eggplant, peppers, citrus fruits, whole grains, berries

Component: Plant sterols (vitamin D precursors)

Disease-fighting Properties: Has anti-cancer properties

Food Sources: Broccoli, cabbage, cucumbers, squash, yams, tomatoes, eggplant, peppers, soy products, whole grains

Component: Potassium
Disease-fighting Properties: Helps to prevent excess sodium and fluid retention; decreases strokes, night cramps, and heart arrhythmia
Food Sources: Bananas, broccoli, cantaloupe, citrus fruits, dried apricots, lima beans

Component: Quercetin
Disease-fighting Properties: Lowers cholesterol, has antioxidant properties; has antiviral and antibacterial effects
Food Sources: Broccoli, onions, tea

Component: Vitamin C
Disease-fighting Properties: Has strong antioxidant properties; helps to prevent cancer; helps to eliminate toxins and heavy metals from the body; may reduce levels of LDL cholesterol while increasing HDL cholesterol; aids in the production of antistress hormones; enhances immunity
Food Sources: Asparagus, broccoli, cantaloupe, cauliflower, citrus fruits, leafy green vegetables, kiwis, papayas, strawberries, tomatoes

Component: Vitamin E
Disease-fighting Properties: Has strong antioxidant properties; slows down buildup of smooth muscle cells on artery walls; increases levels of HDL cholesterol; inhibits platelet aggregation; protects against brain and nervous system disorders
Food Sources: Wheat germ, oatmeal, peanuts, nuts, brown rice, leafy green vegetables

cherries, cranberries, raspberries, strawberries), citrus fruits (lemons, limes, and oranges), melons (cantaloupe, honeydew, watermelon), as well as tropical fruits (guava, kiwi, papaya, pineapple, mango, and star fruit).

Strive to eat fruit two to three times a day. If no weight loss occurs, cut back on the amount of fruit you eat. Temporarily restricting your fruit intake can be effective for weight loss.

Eat vegetables at least four to five times a day. Half of your vegetable intake should be in the form of leafy green salad vegetables. Experiment with the wide variety of nutrient-dense lettuces and leafy green vegetables available such as arugula, baby leaf, red leaf, Bibb, Boston, endive, escarole, frisee, romaine, raddichio, spinach, and watercress. The other half of your vegetable intake should be made up of a variety of vegetables like asparagus, avocado, bamboo shoots, bean sprouts, beet greens, broccoli, Brussels sprouts, cabbage, carrots, cauliflower, celery, chard, cucumber, eggplant, kale, kohlrabi, mushrooms, okra, onion, green peas, peppers, pumpkin, snow pea pods, squash, string or wax beans, summer squash, sweet potato, tomato, turnips, water chestnuts, yams, and zucchini. Corn and white potatoes have a dramatic effect on blood sugar levels and should be eaten sparingly.

Choose organically grown produce, whenever possible. The pesticides, antibiotics, and hormones that are used to produce fruits and vegetables can contribute to a wide range of diseases and overall ill heath. When eating fresh produce raw, leave on the skin (if organic) as it contains many phytochemicals. Try and select seasonal fresh fruits and vegetables, and avoid all frozen and canned produce. Canned fruits and vegetables usually contain large amounts of sugar, salt, and other additives. When preparing vegetables, cook them briefly in a steamer or sauté them lightly. Many important vitamins, minerals, and phytochemicals are sensitive to heat and can be damaged or destroyed by cooking.

Recommended amount: Fruits, two to three times a day; vegetables, four to five times a day.

Whole Grains

Whole grains are an important source of fiber, protein, vitamin E, the B vitamins, and minerals. The fiber found in whole grains binds with cholesterol-producing substances and helps to eliminate them from the body; B vitamins facilitate homocysteine metabolism; vitamin E helps to prevent LDL cholesterol from oxidation. The essential heart minerals magnesium, selenium, copper, and manganese are found in the bran layer of many grains. And because whole grains are complex carbohydrates, they are digested and converted into blood sugar very slowly.

Numerous studies have found that eating more whole grains significantly lowers your risk of heart disease. One study reported in the *Journal of the American Medical Association* followed the whole grain intake of 68,782 women participating in the Nurses' Health Study over ten years. Those who ate the most whole grains (an average of 2.5 servings a day) had half the risk of heart attack or death from coronary heart disease compared to those who ate the least, about one serving a week. Even when other factors were considered, these women still had a lower risk.

There are a wide variety of whole grains to choose from, including amaranth, barley, brown rice, bulgur, buckwheat, kasha, matzoth, millet, oats, quinoa, spelt, teff, and triticale, as well as whole wheat. While whole wheat is the dominant grain used in grain products like bread, crackers, flours, pastas, and cereals, many of the other grains, once rare, are becoming easier to find. For store-bought breads made with white flour, look for soy-based bread, high-gluten bread, or sprout or grain bread. When buying whole-grain products, be sure that the whole grain is used, which ensures that its nutritional content remains.

Eat for Color Diversity

Because no one fruit or vegetable can contain all of the heart-healthy compounds you can benefit from, it's a good idea to make sure you choose from a variety of fruits and vegetables. Aim to eat at least one fruit or vegetable on most days from each color of the rainbow.

Red: Red apples, beets, red bell peppers, cherries, red cabbage, cranberries, red currants, pink grapefruit, red plums, pomegranates, radishes, raspberries, rhubarb, strawberries, tomatoes, watermelon

Orange: Apricots, carrots, cantaloupe, kumquats, sweet potatoes, pumpkin, mangoes, nectarine, oranges, papayas, peaches, persimmons, tangerines, sweet potatoes, pumpkins, winter squash, yams

Yellow: Acorn squash, artichoke, bamboo shoots, bananas, bean sprouts, yellow bell peppers, cabbage, cauliflower, celery root, corn, cucumber, garlic, golden apples, yellow grapefruit, guava, leek, lemons, onions, mushrooms, parsnips, pears, pineapple, potato, rutabaga, star fruit, summer squash, turnips, water chestnuts, wax beans, yellow squash

Green: Alfalfa sprouts, green apples, asparagus, arugula, avocado, beet greens, green bell peppers, bok choi, broccoli, Brussels sprouts, cabbage, celery, Chinese cabbage, collards, green grapes, green peas, herbs (all), kale, kohlrabi, honeydew melon, kiwi, lettuces (all), limes, okra, snow peas, spinach, string beans, Swiss chard, turnip or mustard greens, watercress, zucchini

Blue: Blueberries, Concord grapes, kelp, loganberries

Indigo: Blackberries, black cherries, black currants, boysenberries, plums

Violet: Eggplant, figs, passion fruit, purple grapes, purple plums

Most of the grains consumed in the typical American diet are processed and refined. In fact, 80 percent of Americans eat less than one serving of whole grains a day. All refined flour products such as bread, bagels, crackers, processed cereals, pasta, white rice, instant types of oatmeal and other hot cereals should be avoided, especially if you need to lose weight. These processed foods contain large amounts of simple carbohydrates that surge into your bloodstream, rapidly shooting up your blood sugar.

If you bake, instead of using refined white flour, try substituting almond flour, flaxseed meal, soy flour, soy protein, whole-wheat flour, oat bran, oat flour, spelt flour, or wheat gluten (the protein component of wheat to which many people are sensitive).

Recommended amount: Three times a day.

Meat and Poultry

Meat and poultry are excellent sources of complete protein and important vitamins and minerals. Complete protein foods provide all of the essential amino acids that the body needs to make new protein. The body uses this protein for growth and development, energy, the synthesizing of hormones, enzymes, antibodies (substances that combat viruses), and other substances vital to normal body function.

Although meat and poultry provide the full range of essential amino acids, they are high in cholesterol and saturated fat, which the liver converts to cholesterol. Large amounts of saturated fats are found in red meats (beef, lamb, pork, veal), in the skin of poultry, and in other fatty meats such as bacon, sausage, pork, and organ meats. Meat consumption accounts for 33 percent of the saturated fat in the American diet.

Eat lean red meat only on occasion and limit your consumption of chicken, turkey, or duck (skinned) to several times a week. Avoid all meat and poultry that is smoked, pickled, or processed (luncheon meat, hot dogs, bologna, and others) and in which sugar, monosodium glutamate (MSG), corn syrup, cornstarch, flour, pickling nitrates, or other preservatives are used in preparation. In addition, whenever possible, select meat and poultry that contains no artificial ingredients, is minimally processed, and was raised without the use of artificial growth hormones, antibiotics, or animal byproducts in the feed. Instead rely on other, more healthful, sources of complete protein such as fish, eggs, and legumes, or a combination of incomplete protein foods that meet the body's daily protein requirements.

Recommended amount: Two to three times a week; limit red meat to once a week.

Fish

Fish is a complete protein and a primary source of protein on the Rainbow Diet. Fish (especially cold-water fish such as bluefish, cod, haddock, halibut, mackerel, salmon, sardines, snapper, and trout) are high in omega-3 fatty acids, a polyunsaturated fat. Eicosapentaenoic acid (EPA) and docosahexaenoic acid (DHA) are two omega-3 fats that have been singled out for their powerful heart- and brain-protective properties.

In a landmark study, Eskimos in Greenland and Iceland were studied for their remarkably low rates of heart disease despite a high-fat diet. An inverse relationship was found between fish consumption and mortality rates from heart disease. Those who consumed 30 grams or more of fish a day—that's 20 grams less than the recommended intake in the United States—had a 50 percent lower cardiac mortality rate than those who did not. Since then dozens of studies have shown the ability of fish oil to prevent heart attacks and sudden cardiac deaths by regulating blood pressure, blood clotting, and heart function. One study showed that this lower incidence of cardiac death extended to individuals who ate as little as one or two servings a week compared to those who ate no fish. A diet high in fish as compared to one high in cold cuts or meat is associated with lower harmful LDL cholesterol, lower blood pressure, lower triglycerides, and higher levels of protective HDL cholesterol.

Fish oils produce such dramatic results in a number of ways. The oil in fish has been found to reduce high levels of total cholesterol and trigylcerides, lipoproteins (fat plus protein), and apolipoproteins (highly inflammatory cholesterol particles) in the bloodstream, to promote the production of beneficial HDL cholesterol, and the relaxation of smooth muscles (hence preventing arteriosclerosis and high blood pressure). Fish oil also helps to dilate arteries and inhibit inflammatory substances that constrict them, further contributing to the prevention of high blood pressure.

Fish oils further benefit the heart and cardiovascular system by stimulating the production of substances called prostaglandins. Prostaglandins are powerful hormonelike molecules that control the functioning of many of the body's systems, including the circulatory system, heart, reproductive system, and the immune and central nervous systems. These substances are generally characterized as either inflammatory or inflammatory-reducing in nature.

Series-1 and series-3 prostaglandins (PGE1 and PGE3) are made from quality sources of omega-6 fatty acids and from omega-3 fatty acids, respectively. These two types of prostaglandins act as anti-inflammatories. They reduce pain and swelling, inhibit platelet aggregation, making blood less likely to form into clots and to cause a stroke or heart attack, and they dilate arteries. Another type of prostaglandin—called series-2 prostaglandins (PGE2)—is derived from arachidonic acid, a harmful type of omega-6 fatty acid that is produced from the oxidation of various lipids and fatty acids. Omega-6 fatty acids are found mainly in vegetable oils, margarine, and processed foods. Series-2 prostaglandins are highly inflammatory substances that constrict blood vessels, encourage blood platelets to clot and inflame plaque, making it more likely to burst. All of these conditions set into motion a cascade of biochemical events, which raise your blood pressure and block your body's arteries. Researchers have noted that people with angina often show a lower ratio of EPA to arachidonic acid.

What you eat has a direct effect on which type of prostaglandins are dominant in the body. PGE2 prostaglandins are overproduced when the body does not get enough omega-3 fatty acids. In general, the American diet is low in omega-3s and overly abundant in omega-6 fatty acids. Our overemphasis on processed foods and the underconsumption of cold-water fish and unprocessed oils create an abundance of inflammation-producing prostaglandins (PGE2s) and insufficient amounts of the anti-inflammatory substances (PGE1s and PGE3s).

In addition to fresh cold-water fish or fish oil supplements, omega-3 fatty acids are available from flaxseed, walnuts, and canola and unhydrogenated soybean oils.

Avoid all fried fish, salted and pickled fish, or fish packed in oil. Eat bass, tuna, swordfish, and shellfish (a possible source of hepatitis) infrequently as they can contain high concentrations of pollutants such as heavy metals (particularly mercury) and PCBs (polychlorinated biphenyls). Similarly, select seafood that is either wild-caught or sourced from aquaculture farms where environmental concerns are a priority.

Recommended amount: Daily—even twice a day if you can. Aim to eat fish a total of seven to fourteen times a week.

Beans and Legumes

Beans and legumes can be used as a supplemental source of protein for people who eat animal foods, or they can serve as a high-quality meat substitute for vegetarians. Most vegetable proteins are incomplete. Eating different sources of incomplete protein together makes up for complete protein. In addition to being a source of complex carbohydrates and quality protein, beans and legumes have plenty of fiber and folic acid. They have been shown to help lower cholesterol levels and stabilize blood sugar.

Soybeans are one of the few plant proteins that contain all the essential amino acids found in animal protein. A study in the *American Journal of Clinical Nutrition* found that when people with high cholesterol and triglycerides consumed soybeans and soy products in place of animal protein, their risk of heart disease was lowered due to reductions in total cholesterol, triglycerides, oxidized LDL, homocysteine, and blood pressure.

In addition to soybeans and products made from them, such as soy-

Vegetarians Take Heed

People who are vegetarians tend to have lower blood pressure than meat-eaters. In one well-known study comparing Seventh-Day Adventists, who are lacto-vegetarians—meaning their diets contain eggs and milk but no meat—with omnivorous Mormons, the lacto-vegetarians had lower blood pressure, even after adjusting for the effects of weight. Theoretically the groups were matched for effects of religiosity and abstention from alcohol, tobacco, and caffeine. The study found that long-term adherence to a vegetarian diet was associated with less of a rise of blood pressure with age and a decreased prevalence of hypertension. The study, however, did not clarify the specific body functions or nutrients affected by such a diet.

Apart from religious, social, or ethical reasons for abstaining from eating meat and meat products, a vegetarian diet is not optimal for your health. Vegetarian diets tend to be deficient in nutrients important for the heart and cardiovascular system.

Complete protein foods such as meat, poultry, and fish all contain concentrated sources of vitamins A, E, and B complex and are loaded with iron, zinc, and other nutrients. Vegetarian diets, on the other hand, can lead to vitamin B_{12} and vitamin D deficiency. Studies have shown that children, two years old or younger who are raised as vegetarians, may be shorter and lighter than other children, possibly the result of zinc and calcium deficiencies. Foods such as beans, legumes, and grains—often staples for vegetarians—are high in phytates, substances that cause the elimination of zinc, calcium, and other minerals in the digestive system. A vegan diet that excludes meat, dairy, and eggs is well below recommended calcium requirements for females. Lacto-ovo vegetarians, on the other hand, appear to have less deficiency in zinc, calcium, and vitamin D. Moreover, several studies have suggested that the consumption of at least some animal protein may be necessary for stress resistance; it appears that true vegetarians cannot adapt to stress as well as meat-eaters for lack of nutritional advantages.

While there are many advantages to a vegetarian diet—the likelihood of increased consumption of fresh whole foods and all the nutritional benefits they have to offer, and decreased consumption of refined carbohydrates and junk food, for example—it is our belief that diets such as the Rainbow Diet, which are high in vegetables and fruits and moderate in whole grains and lean animal protein is best for optimal health.

milk, tempeh, and tofu, there are a wide variety of quality beans from which to choose, including chick peas, lentils, soybeans, split peas, and any of the following beans: adzuki, anasazi, black, fava, kidney, lima, mung, or navy beans.

Recommended amount: One to two times a day, or a minimum of five to six times weekly.

Eggs

In spite of the almost universal advice to limit the consumption of eggs because of their high cholesterol content, we think it is good to eat eggs. The egg is a nearly perfect amino-acid food. It provides top-quality protein, is low in saturated fat, rich in protein and cancer-fighting vitamin A, low in calories, high in folic acid and vitamin B_{12}, plus various other B vitamins and trace elements. The egg's cholesterol content is largely modified by its high content of lecithin. Lecithin is a natural emulsifier, that is, it helps to liquefy fat inside the blood vessels and stop plaque build-up. Eggs are not only an acceptable food, they are an essential and valuable addition to a nutritionally well-balanced diet. To consider cholesterol content only is misleading; the ratio of cholesterol to other nutrients is what is important.

There are many conflicting reports regarding the egg's complicity in elevated cholesterol. Despite the fact that each egg yolk contains 200 milligrams (mg) of dietary cholesterol, the latest studies do not indicate a significant positive correlation between egg consumption and increased cholesterol levels. In one typical study, 168 volunteers consumed a reduced-fat diet with an increased polyunsaturated-to-saturated fat ratio. Half the group consumed two eggs a week, while the other half ate seven eggs. After four weeks, testing showed no significant rise in the serum cholesterol levels of the high egg-consuming group. A one-year trial showed that serum cholesterol correlated to saturated fat consumption and not to dietary cholesterol in eggs, as most would have expected.

The overall rate of dietary cholesterol intake in the United States has dropped from 800 mg a day to less than 500 mg a day in the last ten years. At the same time, consumption of the "good" unsaturated fats found in polyunsaturated and monounsaturated oils has increased by 60 percent. These changes in diet have done more to reduce heart disease than all medical procedures combined. These changes in cholesterol consumption have come mainly from the reduction in meat intake, which is 40 percent less than ten years ago. In contrast, egg consumption has dropped only 12 percent, so it is apparent that the reduction in eggs has made little contribution to the decrease in heart attacks.

Did you know that a 100 mg cholesterol intake per day only raises your serum cholesterol by an insignificant 4 mg a day? Dietary saturated fatty acids are the main culprits (along with refined carbohydrates) in serum cholesterol elevation, not dietary cholesterol. Taking supplements of fish oil, primrose oil, niacin, and other nutrients, which you'll learn about in the next chapter, do more to lower cholesterol than the elimination of eggs from the diet. Stress reduction is also an important factor.

The egg is a good source of protein. Most foods contain a lower quality of protein than the egg. The egg is proportionally the most balanced and best source of essential amino acids. In most food, only one or two essential amino acids are deficient or totally lacking, and these are called the "limiting amino acids" for that food. The protein in that particular food will be usable by the body only to the extent that the limiting amino acid is present in another food being ingested at the same time. The egg's superior balance of amino acids makes its protein more usable than those of most other foods.

Careful study of the effect of egg proteins on plasma amino acids shows that egg, like steak, raises the amino acids lysine, valine, threonine, and leucine to extremely high levels. Yet, the ratio to other amino acids is slightly better balanced with the egg than with steak. For example, steak increases the plasma valine-to-plasma methionine ratio to more than five-to-one, while for eggs it is only four-to-one. The egg is slightly better balanced, but not perfectly balanced. Amino acid formulas for supplements are now being studied that may suggest ways to achieve a more balanced rise in plasma amino acids than food itself can provide. At present, however, the egg is your best bet.

Recommended amount: One a day, or up to seven a week.

Dairy Foods

Cheese, milk, and yogurt are complete proteins and are rich sources of calcium and other nutrients. Yet nearly all whole-milk dairy products are high in saturated fat and sodium, which raise harmful LDL cholesterol and increase your risk of heart disease, not to mention calories. Exclude whole-milk dairy products such as milk, cream, butter, cheese, and other foods derived from animals (like ice cream!) from your diet. Instead drink low-fat, fat-free, or skim milk, soy or rice milk. Choose low-fat or fat-free versions of cheeses, sour cream, unsweetened yogurt, buttermilk, and other dairy foods. This way you benefit from the nutrients, but without the fat.

What about butter and margarine? Avoid both. Butter is dense in calories and saturated fat. Margarine, a vegetable shortening often used as a substitute for butter because it is lower in saturated fat and has no cholesterol, contains dangerous compounds called trans fatty acids. Now believed to be much worse than saturated fat, these substances are created during a chemical process known as hydrogenation during which liquid oil is made semi-solid or solid at room temperature. This process generates large numbers of cell-damaging free radicals, which can raise your cholesterol. In addition, trans fats raise LDL cholesterol, decrease beneficial HDL cholesterol, and promote the production of inflammatory series-2 prostaglandins. Trans fats are found in many margarines, vegetable shortenings, and baked goods and processed foods made with these fats. Avoid products that list hydrogenated or partially hydrogenated oils on the label.

Whenever suitable substitute olive oil, a healthy monounsaturated fatty acid, in place of butter. Most unsalted margarines available in natural food stores are made with plant sterols, which are an acceptable substitute for their conventionally prepared counterparts.

Recommended amount: Four times a week or a maximum of one to two times a day of low-fat, fat-free, or skim-milk dairy products, and/or soy or rice milk.

Fats (Oils)

Contrary to public perception, the body needs fat to maintain health. Fat is necessary for brain development in infancy and provides energy and promotes growth throughout life. The typical American diet, however, contains too much of the harmful kind of fat (saturated fats), and not enough unsaturated healthy fats (polyunsaturated and monounsaturated fats). The differences between these oils are based on the number of hydrogen atoms in their chemical structure and in the ways they act within the body.

No amount of saturated fat is good for the heart and arteries. Limiting or avoiding red meat and full-fat dairy products will significantly reduce your risk. Coconut oil and palm kernel oil are also high in saturated fatty acids, so avoid products that contain them. (See Table 4.3 on page 55 for tips on how to reduce the harmful fats from your diet.)

Monounsaturated and polyunsaturated fats, on the other hand, have been shown to have beneficial effects on cholesterol when consumed in moderation. Monounsaturated fatty acids are considered very healthy fats. As mentioned earlier, one of the best sources of monounsaturated fats is olive oil; 74 percent of olive oil contains this good fat. The next-best sources are canola and peanut oils. Monounsaturated oils, especially olive oil, are an important staple in the diets of people living in Mediterranean regions, who have been shown to have low rates of heart disease. Studies have shown that these fats not only reduce levels of harmful LDLs, but also can raise levels of beneficial HDLs. Polyunsaturated fats are most abundant in vegetable oils such as safflower and sunflower oils and in fish oil. These fats lower your total cholesterol, but if eaten in excess, have a tendency to reduce your beneficial HDL cholesterol as well.

Because cholesterol and triglycerides are fats, the "good" monounsaturated and polyunsaturated fats and oils have a particular affinity for cleaning out the bad ones from the body. In addition to their effect on cholesterol, monounsaturated and polyunsaturated fats can benefit those who have high blood pressure. It is thought that these fats work as natural diuretics, thus easing the stress on the blood vessels.

Recommended amount: Three to four tablespoons of any of the following oil or oils: olive, fish, flaxseed, safflower, and sunflower.

Nuts and Seeds

Most nuts and seeds are high in protein, essential fatty acids, and healthy unsaturated fats (good for lowering cholesterol) and abundant in minerals such as magnesium, potassium, calcium (good for lowering blood pressure). But because of their high-fat content, nuts and seeds should be consumed in small quantities. Walnuts, almonds, and pecans contain slightly less fat than other nuts and seeds. For this reason, hyptertensives who are overweight should limit their selection to these nuts.

Avoid salted and roasted nuts. Choose raw, organic, unsalted nuts whenever possible.

Recommended amount: One-fourth cup (approximately one fistful) five to six times a week.

Sugar and Sweeteners

In the last several years sugar has come to be regarded as a major contributor to the development of cardiovascular disease. Eating large quantities of sugary foods and refined carbohydrates triggers the pancreas to release insulin, a hormone that controls how your cells use sugar. If exposed to frequent overdoses of sugar and simple carbohydrates, these cells eventually lose the capacity to respond appropriately to insulin. The pancreas keeps producing insulin, which raises the unused insulin levels higher and higher. Elevated insulin increases cholesterol and triglyceride levels, increases blood pressure, and inflammation in the blood vessels.

TABLE 4.3. TRIMMING THE FAT

Another simple way to trim the fat (and keep your cholesterol down) is to substitute the following low-fat foods in column 2 for the high-fat ones in column 1.

INSTEAD OF:	SUBSTITUTE:
Avocado	Cucumber, zucchini, lettuce
Bacon	Chicken or Canadian bacon
Beef, ground	Lean beef with all fat trimmed, eye of round, top round
Bologna, frankfurter, sausage	Chicken or turkey, lean, thinly sliced
Butter, margarine	Olive, safflower, or sunflower oil
Cream	Evaporated skim milk
Egg, fried	Poached or baked egg
Hot fudge sundae	Frozen yogurt or ice milk with sliced or crushed fruit
Ice cream	Ice milk, frozen low-fat yogurt
Liver	Lean meat, chicken, fish
Milk, whole or condensed	Fat-free, low-fat, or skim milk; soymilk; rice milk
Peanuts	Fruits or vegetable snack
Pork (spare ribs, ground pork)	Well-trimmed lean pork, lean tenderloin, sirloin, or top loin
Salad dressing	Reduced-calorie salad dressing, vinegar, lemon juice
Soft or high-fat cheeses	Low-fat or fat-free cheese, cottage cheese, feta, or mozzarella
Sour cream	Non-fat yogurt, fat-free sour cream
Snack crackers, chips	Brown rice crackers, whole wheat crackers, soy crackers

Sucrose, also known as table sugar, is found predominantly in cane sugar and to a lesser extent in some fruits and vegetables. Americans, in particular, consume huge amounts of sugar—nearly 150 pounds a year per person—most of which comes from refined processed foods. At high levels of refined carbohydrate consumption (50 to 80 percent), increases in blood pressure are observed. A diet high in refined carbohydrates has also been shown to induce sodium retention, and through this retention of sodium, to raise blood pressure. It also depletes potassium from the body. In addition, foods high in refined simple sugars typically are high in saturated fat (which increases cholesterol and weight) as well as salt—all factors that contribute to high blood pressure and heart disease.

People with high blood pressure are frequently found to have insulin resistance, especially when the condition is treated with diuretics. Insulin resistance occurs when cells become resistant to accepting insulin. Insulin resistance, obesity, and blood pressure are tightly interrelated, so an imbalance in one will cause problems in the others. All three are major risk factors for heart disease.

Eliminate all refined sugars from the diet. This includes white, brown, or raw cane sugar, corn syrup, and fructose. Use minimally processed natural sugars sparingly such as honey, maple syrup, molasses, sucanat, barley malt and brown rice syrup. These natural sugars contain beneficial nutrients, and have a very minimal effect on blood sugar.

Sugar substitutes such as sucralose (Splenda), aspartame (Equal, Nutrasweet), and acesulfame K (Sunette, Sweet One, and Sweet 'n Safe) are also an option. Sucrulose is heat stable and works well for sugar-free baking. Low-calorie sugar alcohols such as sorbitol, maltitol, mannitol, and xylitol are natural sweeteners. Their chemical structure makes them mostly indigestible and keeps them from affecting blood glucose the way natural sugar would. In some people, sugar alcohol can produce intestinal side effects precisely because they are not digested well; if such is the case for you, discontinue its use. We find that most people tolerate sucralose well. Herbal sweeteners such as Stevia (classified by the FDA as a supplement) and Lohan (Sweet and Slender) are also good alternatives to consider. Learn which one you like and buy it religiously. The Rainbow Diet includes fewer sugary foods than in the average American diet.

Recommended amount: Use sparingly; no more than two to three times a day.

Seasonings

Many herbs have long been used as culinary spices and for medicinal purposes. Many have been used to treat heart disease and circulatory problems, but only recently has scientific research begun to hone in on the active compounds that make some so valuable. Turmeric, garlic, onion, ginger, and cayenne are particularly valuable for the cardiovascular support they provide.

Turmeric is an herb that is widely used in curry and other Indian dishes. In recent animal studies, curcumin, the main bioactive compound found in turmeric and the ingredient responsible for turmeric's characteristic canary yellow color, was shown to possess numerous cardioprotective properties. Curcumin contains powerful antioxidant properties, which make it particularly effective against the most common form of free radical called reactive oxygen species. The reactive oxygen species neutralized by this herb are xanthine oxidase, superoxide anion, malondialdehyde, glutathione peroxidase, and lactate dehydrogenase. Curcumin also appears to protect against the oxidative stress injury that follows a stroke and stops the oxidation of LDL cholesterol.

Garlic helps the heart and cardiovascular system in many ways. This herb lowers blood pressure through the actions of one its components, allylic sulfide, which dilates blood vessels. It thins the blood by inhibiting platelet aggregation, which reduces the tendency of blood platelets to stick together and inhibits blood clot formation. It can slightly lower total cholesterol and triglyceride levels while increasing the beneficial HDL cholesterol. As a free-radical scavenger, garlic helps prevent the oxidative reactions that promote atherosclerosis. Additionally, it appears to protect the enzymes in the cells lining the arteries that produce nitric oxide, a molecule essential for relaxation of the blood vessels, which helps the body to maintain normal, healthy blood pressure. According to an article in the *Journal of Hypertension,* findings from seven studies on garlic's effects on high blood pressure showed that 600 to 900 mg of garlic a day (equivalent to two to three garlic cloves) lowered systolic blood pressure from 7.7 to 11.1 points and diastolic pressure by 5.0 to 6.5 points.

Like garlic, onions contain large amounts of allylic sulfide. Onions help lower your blood pressure and LDL cholesterol, prevent blood clots, and improve your circulation. Onions are also the richest source of quercetin, a flavonoid that acts as a powerful antioxidant. One of the most impressive studies highlighting the cardioprotective properties of onions is research involving more than 5,000 Finns, who have the highest rates of heart disease in the world. Investigators found that those who had the lowest dietary intake of flavonoids had the highest risk for heart disease, even after factors such as cigarette smoking, high blood pressure, elevated cholesterol and excess weight were controlled for.

Cayenne, also known as chili pepper, has mild blood-thinning properties. Studies have shown that it reduces the formation of blood clots by inhibiting the production of substances known as thromboxanes, which promote the clotting of blood. Studies conducted in cultures where hot chilies are regularly consumed, such as in New Guinea, Bantu, Korea, East Africa, and Thailand, have found its peoples to have the lowest incidence of blood clots in all the world. (*Note:* A small fraction of people may get arthritislike symptoms from consuming chili peppers.) Cayenne, like the other herbs and spices mentioned here, is a rich source of antioxidant protection against free radicals. It also appears to reduce cholesterol by enhancing an enzyme in the liver responsible for metabolizing fat.

Recommended amount: Use liberally each day. Spices and herbs enhance the taste of food, and are often an effective substitute for salt.

Salt

Although salt (sodium) has a bad name, you cannot exist without it. Sodium contributes to the maintenance of normal fluid levels, healthy muscle function, and proper acidity (pH) of the blood. To keep these processes running smoothly, the body requires only small amounts of sodium—1 gram per day—much less than the 10 to 12 grams (two teaspoons) in the average American diet. The hazards of a high-sodium diet go beyond high blood pressure; excess salt in the diet can aggravate many conditions, including premenstrual syndrome (PMS), certain types of kidney disease, and heart failure.

An excess intake of salt attracts water and causes fluid retention in the tissues of the body. This extra fluid expands the volume of blood in your blood vessels, puts pressure on the walls of the vessels, and brings blood pressure up like no other food in such a short period of time.

Being mindful of your salt consumption is essential if you are to control your high blood pressure. Studies and clinical experience have repeatedly demonstrated that reducing salt intake will lower blood pressure in most people. All of our patients are asked to limit their sodium to 2.2 grams or less a day, or to use a table-salt substitute such as high-potassium salt. (Make sure the salt substitute you choose contains only potassium chloride or magnesium chloride, and is not simply "light salt.") Also, as we just mentioned, using herbs and spices can create an abundance of flavor and can help to mask the less salty taste of foods. Cayenne pepper, turmeric, cinnamon, cumin, garlic powder, tarragon, oregano, dill, and parsley are all good alternatives for seasoning food without salt.

Eliminating the use of salt to season your food is a good start, but it's not enough. It is estimated that 80 percent of your salt intake is actually ingested from processed foods. All packaged and prepared foods, canned soups and vegetables (unless marked sodium- or salt-free), ice cream, salad dressings, bread, baking soda, pickles, meat tenderizers (Accent) and meat extenders (MSG, for example) are high in salt. Avoid food products that have *salt, soda, sodium* or the symbol *Na* on the label. Checking the "Nutrition Facts" panel on the label will also help you determine whether the product is low in sodium. Select foods that have a "percent daily value" of sodium of 5 or less, to keep the sodium in your diet to a minimum. For additional ways of cutting back on salt without cutting it out, see Table 4.4 on page 60.

If you find yourself craving salt, supplementing with up to 1,000 mg of magnesium a day may help. The brain controls the appetite for fats and salts. In the case of salt, preliminary investigations indicate that it is regulated by serotonin metabolism. Low levels of serotonin, a mood-lightening neurotransmitter, increase your craving for salt. Supplementing the diet with the amino acids tyrosine, phenylalanine, methionine, and tryptophan has also been found to reduce salt appetite for some people, particularly hypertensives and heart failure patients. Interestingly, researchers have suggested that stress and salt are cyclical, meaning that an increased salt intake produces stress, and craving salt is a sign of stress. Many researchers have shown that decreasing sodium intake can decrease stress. Anything that reduces anxiety, such as a biofeedback, meditation, or exercise, may help to reduce salt cravings. (See Chapter 6 for techniques to help reduce stress.) Thyroid hormone also can reduce salt appetite, if the hormone level is slightly low.

In addition to limiting the amount of salt in your diet, high sodium levels can also be counterbalanced by increasing your potassium intake. As you'll read in the next chapter, a higher ratio of potassium-to-sodium has been shown to lower moderately high blood pressure. In addition to potassium supplements, foods such as bananas, broccoli, chickpeas, acorn squash, spinach, strawberries, and watermelon are rich sources of potassium. Potassium-salt substitutes are another option for decreasing your salt intake.

Recommended amount: 2.2 grams or less per day.

Beverages

Try and limit your consumption of drinks that contain caffeine. This includes tea, coffee, and soda. Caffeine stimulates the brain, raises your stress hormone levels, depletes magnesium and potassium, and elevates blood cholesterol levels and blood pressure. Just two cups of coffee a day can raise blood pressure five or ten points and has been shown to increase coronary heart disease risk by almost 250 percent.

As an alternative, herbal teas are naturally free of caffeine (or else very low in caffeine) and are rich in heart- and artery-healthy minerals, trace elements, vitamins, bioflavonoids, and phytonutrients. Sip one to two cups of any of the following teas daily: barberry, capsicum, comfrey, cramp bark, ginger, green tea, hawthorn, hops, jasmine, mistletoe, parsley, passion flower, skullcap, or valerian. Green tea, in particular, is extremely abundant

TABLE 4.4. SAVING ON SODIUM

INSTEAD OF . . .	SUBSTITUTE . . .	SODIUM AVOIDED
Bologna, 3 ounces (872 mg)	Veal or lamb, 3 ounces roasted (50 mg)	822 mg
Cheese, 1 ounce provolone (248 mg)	Cheese, 1 ounce Swiss (74 mg)	174 mg
Garlic salt, 1 teaspoon (1,850 mg)	Garlic powder, 1 teaspoon (1 mg)	1,849 mg
Kidney beans, 1 cup canned (844 mg)	Kidney beans, 1 cup cooked from dry (4 mg)	840 mg
Oatmeal, 1 envelope instant, ¾ cup cooked (400 mg)	Oatmeal, ¾ cup cooked, old-fashioned or quick (0 mg)	400 mg
Olives, 3 green (242 mg)	Olives, 3 ripe black (96 mg)	146 mg
Sauerkraut, 1 cup, drained (1,121 mg)	Cabbage, 1 cup cooked, shredded (29 mg)	1,092 mg
Soy sauce, 1 tablespoon (892 mg)	Teriyaki sauce or low-sodium soy sauce, 1 tablespoon (630 mg)	262 mg

in polyphenols, a potent group of antioxidants that prevents the oxidation of cholesterol. It is also highly effective at helping curb cravings in those addicted to caffeine. For double-your-pleasure benefits, look for a tea blend that combines two or more of these herbs. Herbal teas can be purchased loose or in tea bags and are available at most natural food stores and herbal mail-order companies.

Decaffeinated coffee, although ulcer-producing, is permitted (up to three 8-ounce cups daily). Diet soda, which is high in caffeine, can be used temporarily to help reduce your appetite for sweets, if needed.

One 8-ounce glass of unsweetened fruit juice a day can be substituted for a piece of fruit, if weight loss is not a problem; or even better, make your own fresh juice. Especially healthy juices are those made from beets, carrots, celery, currant, cranberry, parsley, spinach, and watermelon. Lemon or lime juice can be added to no-salt seltzer with a little sweetener to make lemon- or limeade. Or create your own sodas by adding fresh fruit juice to seltzer.

Recommended amount: Eight 8-ounce glasses of healthy liquids, including water, each day.

Alcohol

Evidence suggests that moderate use of any alcohol, be it beer, wine, or spirits, raises "good" HDL cholesterol and actually protects against heart disease. Moderate use is defined as two alcoholic drinks a day for men and one for women. The bad side effects of alcohol outweigh this one possible good effect, so be cautious about your alcohol consumption. For people with high blood pressure and heart disease, less is better. Drinking three or more drinks a day increases your risk of developing high blood pressure. Excessive alcohol consumption increases the flow of adrenaline, which constricts blood vessels and causes blood pressure to rise. It also may lead to rhythmic disturbances in heart function. Alcohol also acts as a depressant. It may lead to depression in some individuals, which, in turn, can increase carbohydrate consumption, and eventually lead to hypertension. Moreover, alcohol is full of empty calories and easily turns into fat and unwanted weight. Avoid wine made with sulfating agents (food additives commonly used to prevent discoloration of foods).

Recommended amount: No more than three drinks weekly; try substituting your drink with a healthy dessert, especially if you are overweight.

Water

It is important when you have high blood pressure not to drink excessive amounts of water, that is, no more than eight 8-ounce glasses a day. Drink water that is free of impurities. Bottled water is preferable to tap water because your public water supply may contain high levels of chlorine and heavy metals, which are leached from old lead pipes. In general, soft water (water with a low-mineral content) tends to be higher in heavy metals than hard water (water with a high-mineral content) because the lead and cadmium contained in the pipes is dissolved by the soft water, which then becomes a source of these toxic minerals. Studies on lead found the lead content of the ventricles and aorta of heart attack victims to be consistently greater than for normal patients. Most people with heart disease, particularly those living in inner cities, tend to have higher body concentrations of lead, cadmium, and aluminum than people without heart disease. Heavy metals, as you may remember, are associated with an increased incidence of high blood pressure and heart disease. They irritate the lining of the blood vessels, which can lead to inflammation and the formation of plaque.

Of the bottled waters available, we recommend spring water or mineral water. Spring water originates from an underground formation that flows naturally to the surface of the earth. Mineral water contains mineral and trace elements that are in the water from the point of its emergence from a natural source. The natural mineral content in these two types of bottled waters has not been altered.

Recommended amount: Limit your water (and other healthy liquids) intake to no more than eight 8-ounce glasses a day.

TABLE 4.5. THE RAINBOW DIET GUIDE

Use this table as a guide to the foods to avoid and include on the Rainbow Diet. Column 4 provides the amount you should aim to eat from each food category, daily or weekly.

TYPE OF FOOD	AVOID	CHOOSE	AMOUNT PER DAY/WEEK
Alcohol	All wine with sulfites	Beer, spirits, and sulfite-free wine in moderation	No more than three drinks per week unless contraindicated
Beans and legumes	All canned and frozen	All beans cooked without salt	One to two times a day, or at minimum, five to six times a week
Beverages	Caffeinated tea, coffee, and soda	Herbal tea, decaffeinated coffee, diet soda (very little, temporarily), no-salt seltzer, unsweetened fruit juice, fresh fruit and vegetable juices	Eight 8-ounce glasses a day (including water)
Dairy Foods	Cheese spreads, and cheese-food substitutes such as Velveeta; all pasteurized or artificially colored cheese products	Low-fat, fat-free, or skim milk, or soy or rice milk; low-fat or fat-free cheese, including all other cheese byproducts	Four times a week, or at maximum one to two times a day
Eggs	Fried or pickled	Boiled or poached	Up to seven a week
Fish	All smoked or pickled fish, and fish packed in oil	Bluefish, cod, halibut, mackerel, salmon, sardines, snapper, tilipia, trout, sea bass, tuna, swordfish, and shellfish, sparingly	One to two times daily, or seven to fourteen times a week
Fruit	All dried, bottled, canned, and frozen fruit	All fresh	Two to three times a day
Grains	All refined flour products, such as bread, rice, bagels, crackers, processed cereals, pasta, white rice, instant types of oatmeal and other hot cereals	All unrefined grains such as whole wheat, amaranth, barley, brown rice, buckwheat, bulgur, kasha, matzoth, millet, oats, quinoa, spelt, teff, and triticale, as well as their flours in addition to soy flour, soy protein, oat bran, oat flour, flaxseed meal, almond flour, wheat gluten	Three times a day
Meat and poultry	Pork and other fatty meats, including sausage, bacon, hot dogs, and bologna; all smoked, pickled and processed poultry	Chicken and turkey (skinned), red meat, duck (skinned), lamb, and veal, sparingly	Limit red meat to once a week; poultry up to two to three times a week

TYPE OF FOOD	AVOID	CHOOSE	AMOUNT PER DAY/WEEK
Nuts and Seeds	Brazil nuts, cashews, hazelnuts, macadamias, peanuts, pine nuts, pistachios; all roasted and salted nuts	Almonds, walnuts, and pecans; all seeds	¼ cup (approximately a fistful) five to six times a week
Oils (fats)	All saturated fats, trans fats, and hydrogenated and partially hydrogenated fats	Flaxseed oil, safflower oil, sunflower oil, olive oil	Four tablespoons a day
Seasonings	Table salt	All spices	Use liberally
Sweeteners	White, brown, or raw cane sugar, corn syrup, fructose	Honey, maple syrup, molasses, sucanat, barley malt and brown rice syrup; maltitol, mannitol, sorbitol, and xylitol; stevia, lohan; sucralose, acesulfame, or aspartame	Use sparingly, no more than two to three times a day
Vegetables	All canned, bottled, and frozen	All fresh; avocadoes, potatoes and corn, sparingly	Four to five times a day
Water	Tap water	Spring water, mineral water	Eight 8-ounce glasses a day (including other healthy liquids)

RAINBOW-RECOMMENDED MENUS

What follows are two weeks of Rainbow-recommended menus for breakfast, lunch, and dinner. Instead of presenting you with a strict meal plan for each day of the week, the Rainbow Diet menus are grouped by meal with fourteen options to choose from. Because they are interchangeable—as long as you stick to the choices presented for each meal—you have the freedom to eat what strikes your mood that day and yet still receive the nutrients needed for a balanced diet. Have at least two snacks between each meal.

These sample menus are designed for the person with high blood pressure, who also has slightly elevated cholesterol and is overweight. Continue on the diet until your blood pressure, weight, and cholesterol are at healthy levels, then gradually begin to liberalize your diet.

Breakfast Options

Eat breakfast between 7 and 10 A.M. Always have one beverage at breakfast, be it fresh-squeezed orange or grapefruit juice, vegetable juice, caffeine-free green tea or any other herbal tea, or decaf coffee. If desired, sweeten with a sugar substitute or natural sweetener.

Choice #1

1 or 2 soft-boiled or poached eggs topped with a splash of olive oil, balsamic vinegar, and seasonings, and a chopped vegetable of your choice

Choice #2

1 cup fat-free or low-fat plain yogurt with a handful of walnuts, almonds, or pumpkin seeds and berries

Choice #3

1 or 2-egg omelet with some cut-up vegetables of every color (mushrooms, spinach, asparagus, broccoli, and red pepper, for example) cooked in a non-stick pan with water or non-stick cooking spray

Choice #4

$\frac{1}{2}$ cup bran oatmeal topped with a handful of chopped almonds, walnuts, or pecans, $\frac{1}{2}$ cup berries, and 2 to 3 tablespoons unsweetened soy or rice milk

Choice #5

$\frac{1}{2}$ pink grapefruit, sprinkled with 1 teaspoon cinnamon, sugar substitute or natural sweetener
1 poached egg on lightly steamed spinach leaves

Choice #6

$\frac{1}{2}$ cup cantaloupe
1 slice whole-wheat toast with 1 tablespoon almond butter
1 cup unsweetened nonfat or low-fat yogurt

Choice #7

2 egg whites scrambled in a non-stick pan with water or non-stick cooking spray, topped with $\frac{1}{2}$ cup raw or lightly steamed vegetables and seasonings
1 slice whole-wheat toast

Choice #8

$\frac{3}{4}$ cup bran flakes with $\frac{1}{2}$ cup skim milk and $\frac{1}{2}$ cup berries
1 whole-wheat English muffin or bran muffin

Choice #9

1 small whole-wheat bagel or 1 whole-wheat English muffin
   with 1 tablespoon low-fat cream cheese

Choice #10

1 whole-wheat waffle with $\frac{1}{2}$ cup mixed berries

Choice #11

1 slice whole-wheat toast with 1 teaspoon olive oil with
   seasonings

Choice #12

$\frac{3}{4}$ cup bran flakes with $\frac{1}{2}$ cup skim milk, 1 cup berries, and
   a handful of almonds

Choice #13

1 or 2 poached eggs topped with salmon and seasonings on
   whole-wheat English muffin

Choice #14

1 cup berries
2-egg omelet with 1 cup chopped vegetables and seasonings,
   cooked in a non-stick pan with water or non-stick cooking spray

Mid-Morning Snack Suggestions

Snacks should contain some protein in order to keep blood-sugar
levels steady. Here are several suggestions:

- Fat-free or low-fat yogurt with a handful of nuts and berries

- Bananas, plain or with some cinnamon powder or a teaspoon
  of nut butter

- 1 or 2 soft- or hard-boiled eggs with some baby carrots

- 2 ounces low-fat cheese with some grapes, 1 green apple,
  and a handful of unsalted mixed nuts

- 5 whole-wheat sesame seed crackers with dipping sauce of
  olive oil and seasonings

Lunch Options

Eat lunch between 12 and 3 P.M. Always have a drink like fresh-squeezed orange juice, caffeine-free green tea, herbal tea, or other healthful beverage. Sweeten with a little sugar substitute or natural sweetener, if desired.

Choice #1

4–6 ounces warm sardines mixed with 1 cup lettuce and topped with
  1 tablespoon pesto or olive oil with balsamic vinegar and some
  seasonings
$\frac{1}{4}$ cup lightly steamed broccoli

Choice #2

4 ounces water-packed tuna mixed with olive oil and balsamic vinegar
  on whole-wheat bread

Choice #3

1 cup lettuce with a rainbow of colored vegetables such as tomatoes,
  peppers, radishes, and broccoli topped with 1 hard-boiled egg,
  1 slice low-fat cheese, tossed with a dressing of 2 tablespoons
  olive oil, a sprinkling of basil and dill, and a splash of vinegar

Choice #4

6 ounces baked skinless chicken
1 cup spinach leaves with a dressing made of 2 tablespoons olive oil,
  a sprinkling of basil and dill, and a splash of vinegar

Choice #5

6 ounces of poached salmon with herbs of your choice
Salad of 1 cup vegetables of your choice tossed with lemon juice

Choice #6

1 cup homemade chicken soup. If soup is made without pasta,
  have $\frac{1}{2}$ slice of toasted whole-wheat bread

Choice #7

2 cups fat-free or low-fat yogurt mixed with a handful of nuts,
  $\frac{1}{3}$ cup of berries or mixture of $\frac{1}{2}$ cup fruit

Choice #8

4–6 ounces skinless turkey with $\frac{1}{2}$ cup lightly steamed vegetables
  sprinkled with seasonings or a dash of olive oil and balsamic
  vinegar

Choice #9

1 cup homemade vegetable soup
1 slice whole-wheat bread topped with low-fat cheese
1 Granny Smith apple

Choice #10

4–6 ounces skinless barbecued chicken breast
1 cup spinach leaves topped with fresh cranberries tossed with
    1 tablespoon each of olive oil and vinegar

Choice #11

4–6 ounces sliced turkey breast with $\frac{1}{2}$ cup sprouts, 3 slices tomato,
    with 1 teaspoon mustard on whole-wheat pita bread
$\frac{1}{2}$ cup fresh apricots or any other fruit

Choice #12

1–1 $\frac{1}{2}$ cups salad greens with $\frac{1}{2}$ cup garbanzo beans, $\frac{1}{2}$ cup
    yellow corn, 1 ounce walnuts, tossed with $\frac{3}{4}$ tablespoon
    olive oil and 1 tablespoon vinegar

Choice #13

2 slices extra-lean turkey or beef, 1 slice low-fat provolone cheese,
    lettuce, 3 slices tomato, 1 teaspoon mustard on 2 slices
    whole-wheat bread
1 piece of fruit of your choice

Choice #14

2 ounces water-packed tuna, 2 slices tomato, 2 lettuce leaves,
    and 2 teaspoons mustard on 2 slices whole-grain bread
1 orange

Mid-Afternoon Snack Suggestions

🍴 1 cup fat-free or low-fat yogurt with a handful of raisins

🍴 1 slice whole-grain bread wrapped around some turkey breast, tomato, and spinach

🍴 $\frac{1}{2}$ cup unsalted mixed nuts

🍴 1 low-carbohydrate energy bar

🍴 1 Granny Smith apple with 1–2 teaspoons peanut butter on brown rice crackers

Dinner Options

Sit down to dinner between 6 and 8 P.M. Whichever menu you choose, always make sure it contains a fresh rainbow salad tossed with a simple dressing of 3-parts olive oil to 1-part balsamic vinegar. To get the most bang for your nutritional buck, think outside the leaf! Instead of iceberg lettuce, choose romaine, green and red leaf, Boston or Bibb lettuces, add some arugula, escarole, spinach, or watercress and you really up the nutritional content of your salad bowl. "Rainbow" your greens: add chopped vegetables of multi-colors, from radishes and tomatoes to green peppers, avocado, cucumber, and more. Try a salad made of raw broccoli and cauliflower with chopped tomato and olives. Or try diced celery, chopped cabbage, and a little chopped apple for flavor, mixed with olive oil and a dash of sugar substitute or natural sweetener for a yummy slaw that is nutritious, too. When you think salad, think all kinds of yummy raw vegetables, and don't be afraid to throw in some extra stuffers like olives or cubes of leftover meat. The more creative you can get with your salads, the happier and healthier you'll be.

If you're having a late dinner, keep it light. Have some skinless turkey, chicken, fish, tofu, or beans with a fresh salad and a slice of whole-wheat bread. Another light dinner option is a soup with vegetables or chicken and $\frac{1}{2}$ slice of whole-wheat bread. For a beverage, have a glass of skim-, low-fat, or fat-free milk, soy or rice milk, herbal tea, water, no-salt seltzer with lemon, or a glass of wine (but, remember, have alcohol no more than two to three times weekly).

> ## HEART-SMARTS: *Do You Know That . . .*
>
> ➤ The top ten sources of fat in the American diet are hamburgers, meat loaf, hot dogs, ham, lunch meats, whole milk, doughnuts, cakes, cookies, and beef.
>
> ➤ The average American drinks 600 cans of soft drinks a year, each containing seven to nine teaspoons of sugar.
>
> ➤ The avocado is the only vegetable that is high in saturated fat.

Choice #1

6–8 ounces grilled or roasted skinless chicken with $\frac{1}{2}$ cup of brown rice
$\frac{1}{2}$ cup grilled vegetables
Rainbow salad
1 banana sliced and sprinkled with cinnamon or unsweetened cocoa
  powder

Choice #2

2 tablespoons low-sodium tomato sauce on $\frac{3}{4}$ cup cooked whole-wheat
  pasta with 2 to 3 meatballs
Rainbow salad
1 cup low-fat plain yogurt mixed with a handful of berries

Choice #3

4–6 ounces broiled or baked red snapper fillet with lemon juice, topped
  with 1–2 tablespoons of basil pesto
1 cup roasted peppers, carrots, and eggplant
Rainbow salad
Jell-O (available at natural foods stores without artificial ingredients)

Choice #4

4–6 ounces broiled salmon steak or other fish
1 cup lightly steamed broccoli and carrots
Rainbow salad
1 cup low-fat plain yogurt mixed with a handful of berries

Choice #5

Caesar salad made with spinach, celery, and carrots, topped with
   1 boiled egg, 2 ounces low-fat cheese such as mozzarella or feta,
   several sardines or 4 ounces of roasted or grilled skinless turkey
   or chicken tossed with a lemon, mustard, and olive oil dressing
1 apple diced with a handful of walnuts and a touch of balsamic vinegar

Choice #6

4–6 ounces broiled lean steak
1 cup lightly steamed green beans with $\frac{1}{4}$ cup sliced almonds
Rainbow salad
1 cup fresh berries

Choice #7

6 ounces grilled skinless chicken breast
1 cup lightly steamed snow peas
1 baked sweet potato
Rainbow salad
$\frac{1}{2}$ cup steamed pumpkin puree dusted with cinnamon powder

Choice #8

6 ounces grilled, broiled, or roasted red snapper with lemon juice
1 baked sweet potato
Rainbow salad
$\frac{1}{2}$ cup pureed frozen banana topped with $\frac{1}{4}$ cup unsalted mixed nuts

Choice #9

6 ounces roasted skinless turkey
1 cup roasted vegetables of your choice (use non-stick spray)
Rainbow salad
Herbal tea with fresh berries and lemon for flavor

Choice #10

4 ounces broiled salmon or trout
1 cup herb-roasted potatoes (use non-stick spray)
1 cup salad greens with mushrooms and lightly steamed asparagus
   tossed with 1 tablespoon each of olive oil and vinegar
$\frac{1}{2}$ cup strawberries mixed with $\frac{1}{2}$ banana

Choice #11

$^3/_4$ cup cooked whole-wheat pasta topped with 1 cup low-sodium
marinara sauce, 3 ounces chicken or meatballs, and 1 cup diced
vegetables, sprinkled with 1 tablespoon grated low-fat parmesan
cheese
Rainbow salad
Baked apple stuffed with raisins and walnuts

Choice #12

3 ounces roasted skinless chicken breast
$^1/_2$ cup mashed sweet potato
$^1/_2$ cup each lightly steamed carrots and green beans
Rainbow salad
$^1/_2$ grapefruit

Choice #13

4 ounces broiled trout
2 cups lightly steamed green vegetables mixed with $^1/_2$ cup corn
1 cup spinach leaves tossed with 1 tablespoon each of olive oil
and vinegar
Dessert of your choice from one of the other dessert options

Choice #14

4 ounces broiled salmon, stir-fried with 1 cup mixed vegetables
(use non-stick spray)
1 cup cooked couscous
Rainbow salad
Sliced orange

MAKING THE RAINBOW DIET WORK FOR YOU

At first, the Rainbow Diet may represent a large change in your eating habits. Don't expect the transition to be without challenges. Positive change takes time. In Appendix A, we've included several recipes, from smoothies to appetizers to main dishes, to expand your repertoire. Here are a few tips to keep in mind as you traverse your way to a heart-healthy diet.

Food Shopping

Shop from a list. Make reading food labels a habit. Labels provide useful information about serving sizes and ingredients. Choose foods that are low in total fat, saturated fat, cholesterol, and sodium. First eat, then shop. Nothing is more dangerous than shopping when you are hungry. Foods that would never catch your eye when you are in your "right mind" will suddenly look very appealing. Be firm about your choices; do not let others intimidate you to return to old eating habits.

Healthy Cooking

Trim the fat from meat before you cook it. Skin all poultry. Use herbs, salsa, and spices instead of rich sauces, gravies, and extra salt to make food taste good. Bake, broil, roast, or lightly steam foods. Cook with a microwave oven as little as possible. Vegetables and other foods cooked in a microwave lose valuable disease-fighting properties and also undergo changes in their chemical compositions with unknown consequence. Also, carcinogenic toxins may leach from the plastic or paper plates or covers and mix with the food. Do not fry your food. Try non-stick cooking sprays, even water, to cut down on fat.

Do Not Overeat

Eat to live; don't live to eat. It is easy to eat too much. Most people are surprised how much they are actually eating when they weigh or measure their food. If need be, use a measuring cup, measuring spoons or scale to keep track of how much you are eating and what your serving sizes are. Write down what you eat and how much you eat. If it looks like too much, it probably is.

Eat by the Clock

Your body gets hungry every three to five hours. Impulse bingeing is usually the result of poor planning. If you eat at regular intervals and never get too hungry, you will be less likely to overindulge. Always have three meals a day with at least two snacks a day in between. Never skip meals. Once you forego a meal, you will be much hungrier when it's time for the next meal and will likely overeat. Also, missing a meal causes blood sugar levels to drop, which leaves you yearning for processed carbohydrates that deplete your energy even more.

Remember to be selective about the carbohydrates you eat. Avoid foods made of white flour, white rice, and refined sugar. Replace them with brown rice, pasta, and bread made from whole wheat or any other whole grain. If you are intolerant to wheat, replace it with gluten-free products. Choose fiber such as fresh vegetables and fruits, which level off blood sugar. Don't skimp on protein and fat to make room for larger amounts of carbohydrates. Protein and fat give the body energy, help to balance blood sugar, and keep cravings at bay.

Limit your intake of alcohol, fruit juice, and caffeinated drinks. This causes abrupt blood sugar lows, leaving you starved for energy. Also, if you eat sweets on an empty stomach, you'll experience blood-sugar lows, which trigger the desire for more sweets or carbohydrates.

Avoid becoming famished during shopping trips and while traveling. Carry protein snacks such as nuts, low-fat cheese, or hard-boiled eggs. These high-power foods are great when you feel your energy drop. Get enough sleep. When the body and mind are well rested, cravings for carbohydrates often vanish.

Eating for Weight Loss

If you weigh more than is recommended and cannot lose the pounds you wish, cut calories by eating smaller amounts of food. Do not skip meals, just eat less. Eat fewer fats by choosing low-fat foods and cooking with less fat (for suggestions, see Table 4.6 on page 74). Eat more slowly. Take time to taste and savor your food. Get rid of the food in your house that tempts you. Help your pancreas to work better by keeping blood sugar stable. Frequent meals containing protein, fiber, and slow-released carbohydrates from natural unrefined sources help maintain the balance of pancreatic hormones necessary for consistent and ongoing breakdown of fat.

Eat healthy snacks. People who snack between meals find it easier to lose weight because they actually take in fewer calories over the course of a day. Typically, snacks are low-nutrient, high-sugar and high-fat foodstuffs. They contain mostly refined carbohydrates that inhibit the optimal fat-loss environment. Even healthy snacks can be deceiving. Fruits, by themselves, can spike blood sugar and insulin levels. Remember, healthy snacks have to be planned otherwise you will find yourself next to the vending machine.

To lower your carbohydrate intake further, you'll want to severely limit foods with the following ingredients: sugar, sucrose, canned sugar, beet juice, high fructose corn syrup, honey, molasses, bleached refined flour, corn starch and rice flour. Explore lower-carbohydrate substitutes for high-carbohydrate foods, for example: for breadcrumbs, substitute ground almonds, commercial low-carbohydrate bake mix, or commercial low-carbohydrate breading; for mashed potatoes, substitute pureed cauliflower; for French fries, oven-roast sliced carrots with spices; for rice, substitute broccoli grains (put a few broccoli spears in the food processor until the pieces are the size of grains and either stir-fry or steam them); for refined wheat pasta, substitute zucchini noodles (thin strips of zucchini sliced lengthwise and lightly steamed), cabbage noodles, spaghetti squash, commercial-low carbohydrate soy pasta, or small amounts of whole-wheat pasta. Be creative.

TABLE 4.6. WAYS TO SAVE ON CALORIES

Here are suggestions for food swaps to save on calories that add hypertension- and heart disease–boosting pounds. The right-hand column shows the number of calories avoided.

INSTEAD OF . . .	SUBSTITUTE . . .	CALORIES SAVED
Bagel	English muffin (whole-wheat)	60
Whole-wheat bread, 1 slice	Multigrain bread, 1 slice	30
Hamburger with cheese, 4 ounces	Hamburger, 4 ounces	80
Chicken breast half with skin, fried	Chicken breast half without skin, roasted	80
Chow mein or chop suey with noodles (beef), 8 ounces	Chow mein or chop suey with noodles (chicken), 8 ounces	120
Clam chowder (New England), 8 ounces	Clam chowder (Manhattan), 8 ounces	70
Cola, 12 ounces	Cola, diet, 12 ounces	159
Corn kernels, 8 ounces	Broccoli spears, 8 ounces	90
Dressing, Blue cheese, 1 tablespoon	Dressing, low-calorie Italian, 1 tablespoon	70
Frankfurter (beef)	Frankfurter (turkey)	45
Lasagna, frozen, 12 ounces	Lasagna, reduced-calorie, 12 ounces	250
Milk, whole, 8 ounces	Milk, low fat (1 percent), 8 ounces	50
Apple juice, 8 ounces	1 apple	50
Peanut butter, 1 tablespoon	Jam (fruit only), 1 tablespoon	40
Potato, baked with skin	Potato, baked without skin	75
Tortilla, 1 wheat	Tortilla, 1 corn	65
Tuna, 3 ounces oil-packed	Tuna, 3 ounces water-packed	30
1 waffle, 7 inches square	2 pancakes, 4 inches round	85

Eating Out

Don't avoid restaurants to keep your blood pressure and cholesterol down. Food for your heart can be wonderful, not wimpy, and hearty as well as healthy, even if you aren't in the kitchen calling the shots.

Today many restaurants and some diners and coffee shops offer healthy food choices that are low in fat, cholesterol, and calories. If that's not an option, choose a restaurant with a large variety of foods so you will have many choices. Ordering à la carte can provide flexibility in choosing what foods to eat. Also a salad bar allows you a wide range of selections. (Check whether sulfating agents have been used first, however. Sulfites are additives commonly used in restaurants and salad bars to prevent discoloration of foods.) Fast-food restaurants need to be chosen carefully to avoid hidden sources of unhealthy ingredients. It can be difficult to get such establishments to reveal a list of ingredients for the prepared dishes they offer.

Stick to dishes that contain fresh, colorful ingredients that are simply prepared, yet good tasting. Say "no" to all fried foods, cake, pie, ice cream, hamburgers and other fatty meats, mayonnaise, creamy dressings, whole milk or milk shakes. Say "yes" to grilled, broiled, or baked foods, fruits and vegetables, lean meat, poultry and fish, simple vinegar and olive oil dressings, fat-free, low fat or skim milk. Ask your server to replace butter with olive oil, and white bread with whole wheat. Ask that salt not be added during the preparation of your meal and that all sauces be served on the side so you can control how much you are putting on your food.

As for desserts, the healthiest cold desserts are natural Jell-Os, sorbets, fruit ices or glazes. All are fat-free—and better restaurants may prepare them without sugar as well. Keep portions small. Another good meal-ender: fresh berries or melon topped with a dollop of low-fat sour cream in place of whipped cream. Or, for a no-calorie twist, add fresh ginger root, a great contributor to heart health; you will never miss the cream or sugar. Frozen bananas can be whipped in a food processor to make sorbet-type desserts or smoothies, which are great—and great for the heart. Also try natural fruit popsicles. Stick with fruits as the sweetener.

Don't make yourself—or your server—crazy, but do what you reasonably can when ordering to ensure that your meal is a healthier one. Once you've placed your order, have a glass of wine, relax, and enjoy.

You've now learned how to choose the proper foods for lowering your blood pressure and elevated cholesterol. In the next chapter we'll explore how to support these foods with supplements.

CHAPTER 5

Key Supplements for Full-Spectrum Support

The key nutrients that form the core of the supplement plan on the No-More Hypertension and Heart Disease Program are naturally present in those foods abundant in the Rainbow Diet. And while no food supplement can substitute for a wholesome, well-balanced diet, they are an indispensable source of nutritional support. There are several reasons for this.

First, you can't be sure the food that you eat meets your nutritional needs. Farming practices and growing conditions in nutrient-depleted soil, harvesting and shipping practices that have been sped up to cut down on transit time, and improper storage are all real and uncontrollable variables that can compromise the quality of the nutrients in the food you eat. Add to this environmental pollutants, stress, medications, aging, and your own individual biochemistry—all of which can interfere with your body's ability to absorb nutrients—and taking supplements starts to make sense.

Second, supplements contain, in concentrated form, the nutrients found in whole foods. Taking supplements can help you to zero in on a specific problem—such as high blood pressure or heart disease—and in amounts that would be hard to get from diet alone. Think of these supplements as a "rainbow" packed in a pill.

Nutritional supplements have many advantages over drugs. Drugs are foreign to the body. They work by interfering with its natural processes. In contrast, nutritional supplements are substances normally found in the body and work by promoting normal biological processes. Each of the following substances can replace dangerous cholesterol and high blood pressure-lowering drugs with safe supplements that work like drugs, without the health-damaging side effects.

Here are the key nutrients that you'll be taking daily on the No-More Hypertension and Heart Disease Supplement Plan:

- Dr. Braverman's Heart Formula (or the content equivalent in another brand)
- Antioxidant complex (vitamins C and E, selenium, and zinc)
- Amino acids (arginine, carnitine, taurine, methionine/cysteine, and tryptophan)
- Essential fatty acids (fish oils, gamma linoleic acid, flaxseed oil)
- Minerals (potassium, magnesium, calcium, GTF chromium)
- Vitamins (CoQ_{10}, vitamin B_6, niacin, pantethine)
- Garlic, fiber, pectin, and other foods that can be taken as supplements

These supplement stars of the No-More Hypertension and Heart Disease Program have been clinically proven to slow or stop the progression of heart and cardiovascular disease. Using them transforms poor cardiovascular risk profiles and provides valuable nutrients. Blood pressure, cholesterol, triglycerides, and blood sugar go down while magnesium, potassium, HDL cholesterol, and sexual appetite rise! The quantities for each of these substances will vary slightly by person and some nutrients may be added or subtracted and doses adjusted as you progress. Specific directions for using them in combination with the Rainbow Diet are provided in Chapter 7, but for now we'd like to introduce you to this family of nutrients and explain how they do what they do. Table 5.1 below lists the nutrients, their recommended dose range, mode of action, and therapeutic results, including potential side effects at high doses.

TABLE 5.1. THE NO-MORE HYPERTENSION AND HEART DISEASE SUPPLEMENT PLAN		
SUPPLEMENT	**METHOD OF ACTION AND RESULT**	**POSSIBLE SIDE EFFECTS AT HIGH DOSE**
ESSENTIAL FATTY ACIDS		
Fish oil (EPA or DHA, 2–10 grams)	Inhibits production of PGE2 and promotes production of PGE1 and PGE3; dilates arteries; prevents platelets from becoming sticky; lowers triglycerides; raises HDL	Belching, bruising
Gamma-linolenic acid (GLA, evening primrose oil, black currant oil, or borage oil, 1–5 grams)	Inhibits production of PGE2 and promotes production of PGE1 and PGE3; acts as diuretic; reduces LDL cholesterol	Diarrhea

SUPPLEMENT	METHOD OF ACTION AND RESULT	POSSIBLE SIDE EFFECTS AT HIGH DOSE
Linoleic acid (safflower, sunflower, flaxseed oil, 2–20 grams)	Acts as diuretic; reduces LDL cholesterol	Diarrhea
VITAMINS		
CoQ$_{10}$ (30–150 mg)	Increases oxygenation to the heart; improves heart function; has antioxidant properties; prevents LDL cholesterol from oxidizing; lowers the hormones angiotensin and aldosterone, which play a role in controlling blood pressure	Diarrhea
Niacin (vitamin B$_3$, 400 mg–2 grams)	Dilates blood vessels; lowers LDL cholesterol, triglycerides and fibrinogen; increases HDL cholesterol	Flushing, itching
Pantethine (1–2 grams)	Decreases triglycerides	May imbalance other B vitamins
Pyridoxine (vitamin B$_6$, 200 mg–1 gram)	Acts as diuretic; prevents build up of homocysteine	Neuropathy
Vitamin C (2–7 grams)	Acts as powerful antioxidant; protects blood vessels from free-radical damage; inhibits oxidation of LDL cholesterol; dilates arteries; improves circulation; strengthens blood vessel walls; prevents platelet aggregation; helps to detoxify heavy metals; helps metabolize cholesterol into bile acids	Diarrhea, flatulence
Vitamin E (1,600 IU)	Acts as powerful antioxidant; protects blood vessels from free-radical damage; inhibits oxidation of LDL cholesterol; thins blood; prevents platelet aggregation; improves circulation	May elevate blood pressure
MINERALS		
Calcium (1–3 grams)	Increases excretion of sodium; regulates contraction and relaxation in heart muscle inflammation	Constipation, kidney stones,
GTF Chromium (200–1,000 micrograms [mcg])	Prevents myocardial infarction; helps to metabolize glucose and to maintain stable blood sugar levels; aids in fat loss	Flatulence
Magnesium (1–3 grams)	Dilates coronary arteries; improves blood flow to the heart; increases beneficial HDL cholesterol; prevents platelet aggregation; regulates contraction and relaxation in heart muscle; stabilizes heart rhythm	Diarrhea, tetany (muscle contraction), low blood pressure
Potassium (10–30 mg)	Increases sodium excretion; decreases blood volume, important in the proper functioning of the heart muscle; helps to maintain a balanced sodium-potassium ratio in blood vessels	Heart attack, indigestion, ulcer

SUPPLEMENT	METHOD OF ACTION AND RESULT	POSSIBLE SIDE EFFECTS AT HIGH DOSE
Selenium (100–400 mcg)	Has antioxidant properties; inhibits oxidation of fats; helps remove mercury and other heavy metals from the body	Hematuria (blood in the urine)
Zinc (15–20 mg)	Has antioxidant properties; inhibits oxidation of fats; helps remove heavy metals from the body; enhances immune function	Anemia, nausea, neutropenia (low white cell count)
AMINO ACIDS		
Arginine (1–4 grams)	Improves blood flow; decreases cholesterol	Arthritis
Carnitine (1–2 grams)	Transports fatty acids to the heart for energy; removes toxic wastes; improves blood flow; lowers total cholesterol and triglycerides; raises HDLs; improves heart conditions	Diarrhea, flatulence
Methionine (1–3 grams, or cysteine, 2–7 grams)	Breaks down fats; protects blood vessels from free-radical damage; is used to make key anti-oxidants and detoxifying substances	Flatulence
Taurine (1–5 grams)	Decreases total cholesterol; facilitates action of sodium, potassium, calcium, and magnesium; strengthens heart muscle; stabilizes nerve impulses involved in heartbeat; neutralizes heavy metals	Gastritis, flatulence
Tryptophan (3–7 grams, by prescription only)	Used to make serotonin, melatonin, and niacin; alleviates stress; lowers blood pressure and reduces risk of heart attack	Drowsiness
FOOD SUPPLEMENTS		
Garlic (1–2 grams)	Protects blood vessels from free-radical damage; lowers blood pressure; thins the blood; reduces total cholesterol; increases HDL cholesterol	Bad breath, indigestion
Fiber (20–30 grams)	Lowers cholesterol; stabilizes blood sugar; eliminates toxic metals; promotes weight loss	May decrease absorption of calcium, iron, and zinc
Olive oil (2–20 grams)	Reduces LDL cholesterol; increases HDL cholesterol	Diarrhea
Pectin (10 grams)	Lowers LDL cholesterol; eliminates toxic metals	Constipation

ESSENTIAL FATTY ACIDS

Essential fatty acids (EFAs) are the building blocks for all the other fats in your body. Because the body cannot manufacture these essential fats on its own and must obtain them from food and supplements, they are called essential fatty acids.

EFAs can dramatically contribute to health and healing. They are components of the outer membrane of every cell. They help to rebuild and construct new cells. They influence hormone activity, central nervous system function, reproduction, inflammation, immunity, and in the right amounts, are valuable for the production of a group of hormonelike chemicals called prostaglandins. We mentioned these substances briefly in earlier chapters. Prostaglandins play a major role in regulating your blood pressure, heart function, blood platelets, smooth muscle action, and numerous other activities in your body.

Essential fatty acids are primarily derived from two families of fatty acids called the omega-3s and omega-6s. The highest amounts of omega-3 oils are found in cold-water, fatty fish. There is also a vegetable source of omega-3 fat that can be found in flaxseed, and to a lesser degree, in walnuts, soybeans, and pumpkin seeds. Omega-6 oils are derived from both plant and animal sources. Plant sources include polyunsaturated vegetable oils such as safflower and sunflower oils. They are also found in abundant supply in certain plants such as primrose, borage, or black currant seeds, and in some animal foods such as lean meats and organ meats.

Alpha linoleic acid (LNA) heads the omega-3 family of oils, while linoleic acid (LA) heads the omega-6 family. In ideal circumstances, your body is able to convert alpha linoleic acids in omega-3 oils into eicosapentaenoic acid (EPA) and then into docosahexaenoic acid (DHA). The linoleic acid from omega-6 oils can be converted into gamma-linolenic acid (GLA) and arachidonic acid (AA). The EPA and GLA are then converted into beneficial prostaglandins.

As with all nutrients, factors such as poor diet, stress, pollution, aging, and ill-health can inhibit the conversion of alpha linoleic acid and linoleic acid into EPA, DHA, and GLA. By supplementing with direct sources of these essential nutrients, you can circumvent any obstacles to absorption and ensure that you are receiving their cardiovascular benefits directly.

Many studies have shown the ability of these oils to lower blood pressure and cardiovascular risk factors significantly. Hence, all our patients are treated with one of the following: EPA and DHA (fish oil), GLA (primrose oil, borage, or black currant seed oil), or linoleic acid (safflower, sunflower or flaxseed oils)—or, in some cases, all three.

Fish Oil

As stated earlier, fish oil contains omega-3 essential fatty acids, which are excellent sources of eicosapentaenoic acid (EPA) and docosahexaenoic acid

(DHA). Omega-3s in the form of EPA and DHA are found in all fish and seafood, but the higher the fat content of the fish, the better.

As discussed in the previous chapter, Omega-3s EFAs have been found to have many heart- and brain-protective properties. Numerous large-scale studies have shown that the oil in fish significantly lowers blood pressure and other heart disease risk factors. In one of these studies, when a group of seventy-eight people with untreated high blood pressure were given fish oil supplements daily, it caused a statistically significant drop in both systolic and diastolic blood pressure. It has been proven to protect the functioning of the heart and to reduce heart attacks by keeping blood platelets slippery. It works to prevent blood platelet aggregation, and greatly lowers triglycerides and LDL and VLDL cholesterol levels while increasing beneficial HDL cholesterol. Omega-3s also promote production of healthy anti-inflammatory series-3 prostaglandins (PGE3) and inhibit the formation of series-2 prostaglandins (PGE2). Omega-3 EFAs are also used by the body to form brain cells and other parts of the nervous system.

Although the Rainbow Diet recommends eating from seven to fourteen portions of omega-3-rich fish a week, supplementing with fish oil such as cod liver or mackerel oil in doses of up to 10 grams a day is a good idea—especially for people with increased risk of coronary heart disease. If you're a vegetarian, you can get linolenic acid from flaxseed oil. Enzymes in your body convert the linolenic acid in the flaxseed oil into EPA and DHA.

Gamma-Linolenic Acid

Gamma-linolenic acid (GLA) is one of the main fatty acids found in the omega-6 oils. Primrose oil (also known as evening primrose oil), borage oil, and black currant seed oil are quality sources of GLA that are not readily found in foods.

GLA is converted into the prostaglandin called PGE1. Studies have shown that GLA works with PGE3 (derived from EPA) to protect against heart disease by keeping the blood platelets slippery, preventing coagulation, and reducing cholesterol. Studies have shown that these essential fats also function as a diuretic and lower blood pressure. When present in the body in sufficient quantities, PGE1 and PGE3 have a PGE2 inhibitory effect. PGE2, which is derived from arachidonic acid (AA), is inflammatory and appears to trigger platelet aggregation and promote blood platelets to clot. PGE2 also causes the kidneys to retain salt, encouraging water retention.

Dietary fatty acid intake is of particular importance in relation to blood pressure when weight reduction is also called for, as is the case with many of our patients. GLA, in particular, appears to boost metabolism and activate the burning of fat.

Linoleic Acid

Linoleic acid is another main fatty acid found in the omega-6 oils. It is most abundant in polyunsaturated oils such as safflower, sunflower, and flaxseed oil. Dietary supplementation with linoleic acid or other polyunsaturated fatty acids are useful in controlling high blood pressure. It is thought that linoleic acid, in particular, works with an enzyme in the lungs to lower blood pressure. In addition, *cis*-linoleic acid (a modified form of polyunsaturated oils) is easily converted to GLA and eventually to PGE1, which dilates and inhibits platelet aggregation. In other words, it keeps the arteries open and lessens clogging.

VITAMINS

Vitamins promote virtually all biochemical reactions in the body. They are indispensable to normal metabolism and the maintenance and repair of the body. They make enzymes, hormones, energy, new cells, and even DNA. Many vitamins also act as extremely potent antioxidants, and work together as a team to limit the damage caused by free radicals.

Vitamins are classified as either water soluble or fat soluble depending upon the molecule on which they are transported through the bloodstream. Water-soluble vitamins are excreted by the urine and must be replenished daily. The water-soluble vitamins are vitamin C and the B-complex group of vitamins. Fat-soluble vitamins, on the other hand, can remain and work for longer periods of time. These vitamins include vitamins A, D, E, and K.

Scientific studies have found that many people don't consume adequate amounts of vitamins A, C, E, and other nutrients—nutrients essential for a healthy cardiovascular system.

Vitamin E

Vitamin E is the body's principal fat-soluble antioxidant. As an antioxidant, vitamin E prevents LDL cholesterol from reacting with oxygen, thus preventing LDL deposits earlier on in cardiovascular disease from damaging your blood vessel walls. It also protects other fat-soluble vitamins such as vitamins A and D from free-radical damage. Vitamin E slows down the buildup of smooth muscle cells on artery walls, which contribute to plaque. It decreases excessive platelet aggregation, and may increase levels of beneficial HDL cholesterol. It is also a mild anticoagulant (blood thinner).

Studies have suggested that your blood level of vitamin E may be your single, best predictor of heart disease risk. Studies have shown that people with high blood pressure often have low levels of vitamin E, as well as other essential antioxidants. A group of diseases of the heart muscle known as cardiomyopathy, which results in impaired heart function, has also been associated with vitamin E deficiency.

High levels of vitamin E are essential for preventing heart attacks and may even prove to be more important in prevention than monitoring cholesterol. A 1996 study published in the journal *Lancet* showed that when 2,000 people with advanced heart disease took 400 to 800 IU of natural vitamin E (d-alpha tocopherol), their risk of nonfatal heart attack was lowered by 77 percent. These results are more powerful than the results of studies on the benefits of cholesterol-lowering drugs.

An analysis of the five largest trials studying vitamin E's role in heart health, reported in *Current Opinion of Lipidology,* found that supplemental vitamin E reduced the risk of heart attacks in the majority of people with preexisting heart disease.

Studies also show that vitamin E can even protect you from some of the damaging cardiovascular effects of eating a high-fat, high-carbohydrate meal. In one study people ate the same fast-food breakfast on two different days. After eating a meal on the first day without vitamin E supplementation, the arteries reacted by constricting. The next day 800 IU of vitamin E and 1,000 mg of vitamin C were taken along with the breakfast. After that meal, the arteries were relaxed and dilated normally.

Although vitamin E may be most widely known for protecting against heart disease, it also helps protect against Alzheimer's disease and cancer, enhances the immune system, lowers levels of inflammatory prostaglandins (PGE2), slows the aging process, and alleviates other health complaints—from burns to PMS.

Vitamin E, like many of the other important nutrients for the heart and cardiovascular system, is no longer abundant in the typical American diet. In addition, polyunsaturated oils used widely in processed foods may lower vitamin E levels. So it is important to obtain ample amounts of vitamin E (1,600 IU a day) in a diet high in polyunsaturated oils. Significant quantities of vitamin E are found in the Rainbow Diet in brown rice, cold-pressed vegetable oils, cornmeal, dark green leafy vegetables, eggs, nuts, oatmeal, seeds, soybeans, sweet potatoes, watercress, wheat, and whole grains.

The natural form of vitamin E is the most potent and is more available for use by the body. When shopping, look for *d*-alpha-tocopherol (the synthetic form is listed as *dl*-alpha-tocopherol). It's important to note that high levels of vitamin E, ranging from 1,600–2,000 IU, may raise blood pressure slightly and that should be watched.

Vitamin C (Ascorbic acid)

Vitamin C is the body's principal water-soluble antioxidant. It is essential for tissue growth and repair, builds collagen, strengthens weak and damaged arteries, protects against blood clotting, improves blood flow and the dilation of blood vessels in people with atherosclerosis, angina pectoris, congestive heart failure, and high blood pressure. Vitamin C also combines with lead and other heavy metals and helps the body excrete them more quickly. In addition to its antioxidant properties, it is now thought that vitamin C's effectiveness may also be achieved by modulating the activity of a natural chemical in the body known as nitric oxide, which improves circulation.

New studies suggest that vitamin C may actually have a bigger role in preventing coronary heart disease than was previously thought. Research on people taking high levels of vitamin C has shown they exhibit lower total cholesterol and LDL cholesterol, and higher levels of beneficial HDL cholesterol. Vitamin C enhances the conversion of cholesterol to bile acids, which can be easily eliminated by the body. Similarly, low levels of vitamin C are linked to dangerously high levels of cholesterol (hypercholesterolemia) and stroke. A study reported in the journal *Stroke* measured the vitamin C levels of 2,120 people for twenty years and found that those with the lowest levels of vitamin C faced a 70 percent increased risk of stroke than those with the highest levels of vitamin C in their blood.

Numerous studies show that people with high levels of vitamin C have blood pressure readings that are slightly lower than people with lower levels. In one study reported in *Lancet,* thirty-nine patients with mild to moderate high blood pressure took 500 mg of vitamin C or a placebo daily. After one month, the systolic pressures of the people taking vitamin C were lowered by 11 mm Hg, while their diastolic pressures were down 6 mm Hg—a 9 percent decline in blood pressure—significantly better results than for those people taking the placebo.

Vitamin C is found primarily in fruits and vegetables. The Rainbow Diet is rich in food sources loaded with vitamin C, including asparagus, black broccoli, Brussels sprouts, cantaloupe, grapefruit, green peas, kale, lemons, onions, oranges, papayas, pineapple, spinach, Swiss chard, tomatoes, and watercress.

Vitamin C is available in tablets, capsules, chewable tablets, and powder, in both synthetic and natural forms. No one form of vitamin C works better than another. Choose whichever type is most convenient for you.

Coenzyme Q_{10} (CoQ_{10})

Coenzyme Q_{10} (CoQ_{10}) is an antioxidant and vitaminlike enzyme. Its level is ten times higher in the healthy heart than in any other organ in the body. CoQ_{10} helps to produce ATP (adenosine triphosphate), a substance that forms in the mitochondria, the little "powerhouses of the cell." Nearly one-fourth of the cells in the heart muscle are mitochondria, and for good reason. The heart requires substantial amounts of CoQ_{10} to keep pumping blood nonstop through an extensive 60,000-mile network of blood vessels over a lifetime.

Research has found that people with heart diseases tend to be deficient in CoQ_{10}. Low levels of CoQ_{10} have been found in people not only with conditions involving a weak or damaged heart, such as with cardiomyopathy or congestive heart failure, but also in people with high blood pressure. By helping the heart pump blood more efficiently, CoQ_{10} helps to lower blood pressure.

As an antioxidant, CoQ_{10} combines with vitamin E to help prevent LDL cholesterol from oxidizing. It also protects vitamin E from free-radical damage. Cholesterol-lowering drugs (statins) interfere with CoQ_{10} production in the body.

Good sources of CoQ_{10} in the Rainbow Diet include cold-water fish (also high in omega-3 essential fatty acids) such as mackerel, salmon, and sardines. CoQ_{10} is also found in beef, spinach, and peanuts.

Niacin (Vitamin B_3)

A water-soluble B vitamin, niacin has long been recognized as an effective treatment for lowering triglycerides and harmful LDL cholesterol, while significantly increasing beneficial HDL cholesterol and improving circulation. Niacin supplementation is a particularly effective agent against an increased level of LDL in patients with type II hyperlipoproteinemia. Studies have also shown that niacin reduces the average numbers of blood vessel wall lesions per subject and blocks the formation of new lesions.

Large doses of at least one to three grams of niacin a day are needed to be effective. At this dose, niacin can cause a red flush on the skin that, while harmless, may be uncomfortable. That niacin flush, however, may be evidence of the very vasodilating-producing properties that enable it to effectively lower blood pressure.

A 1996 study published in the *Annals of Internal Medicine* compared niacin and the cholesterol-lowering drug lovastatin. After a little more than four months, the group taking the lovastatin had a 32 percent decrease in LDL cholesterol, while those taking the niacin had a 23 percent decrease. But, those in the niacin-taking group benefited from a 33 percent increase in HDL cholesterol, while those in the lovastatin-taking group showed only a 7 percent increase.

About half the body's niacin requirements come from food and the other half is made from the essential amino acid tryptophan, which you can only get from protein foods. Sources of niacin in the Rainbow Diet are broccoli, carrots, dates, eggs, fish, tomatoes, and whole-wheat products.

To prevent niacin's characteristic flush reaction when taking it in supplement form, start at doses of 100 mg twice a day with meals, doubling the dose every three days. If the flush is too great at any dose, cut the next dose by one-half or one-fourth. Zero-flush formulas enable you to start at 800 mg and rapidly increase to 2 to 3 grams. If you still experience discomfort, consider trying one of two other popular supplements for normalizing cholesterol: policosanol, a naturally occurring compound extracted from sugar-cane wax, beeswax, or rice-bran wax; or red rice yeast extract, the fermented product of rice on which red yeast (*Monascus purpureus*) has been grown.

Pantethine (Vitamin B$_5$)

Pantethine is the biologically active form of pantothenic acid (vitamin B$_5$). Pantethine is thought to work by helping to transport useful fatty acids in cells. It lowers total cholesterol, LDL, and triglycerides, while raising protective HDL.

Pyridoxine (Vitamin B$_6$)

Pyridoxine, a water-soluble B vitamin, helps convert the amino acids in the protein you eat into proteins your body uses to make enzymes, hormones, neurotransmitters, prostaglandins, and more. During this process, pyridoxine, in conjunction with the B vitamins folic acid and cobalamin, breaks down a toxic substance called homocysteine, a natural byproduct of protein metabolism. High blood levels of homocysteine can occur when too much protein (especially red meat) is consumed in proportion to inadequate levels of the B vitamins pyridoxine, folic acid, and cobalamin. These three B vitamins are found mainly in high-quality protein such as eggs, fish, poultry, and meat. The higher their levels in the blood, the lower your level of homocysteine. Homocysteine damages blood vessel walls, which in turn, promotes the buildup of cholesterol.

Pyridoxine also inhibits platelet aggregation through its byproduct, pyridoxal 5′ phosphate (a more biologically active form of pyridoxine) and functions as a mild diuretic, which helps to reduce edema (swelling due to the accumulation of fluid in the body's tissues). Conventional diuretics block the absorption of pyridoxine by the body.

Other foods, besides high-quality proteins, that supply pyridoxine include carrots, peas, spinach, sunflower seeds, walnuts, and brown rice and other whole grains—all foods abundant in the Rainbow Diet.

MINERALS

Minerals are divided into two groups: major minerals and trace minerals. The body needs greater quantities of major minerals such as calcium, magnesium and potassium than trace minerals such as chromium, selenium, and zinc, but they are all no less important.

Unlike vitamins, minerals are actually part of the body's tissues and fluids. They are needed for maintenance of the body's fluid balance, for nerve transmission, for muscle contraction, for the formation of blood and bone, and the manufacture of hormones. Minerals are essential for the proper utilization of vitamins, other minerals, and other nutrients. All of these roles are involved in the prevention and treatment of high blood pressure and heart disease.

Like vitamins, it can be difficult to obtain the amount of minerals necessary for cardiovascular health through diet alone. Mineral intake in the typical American diet is often woefully lacking for many of the same reasons that vitamin intake is—poor soil conditions, processing and manufacturing, food preparations, and more. In contrast, the Rainbow Diet is a mineral-rich food plan.

Some minerals are best absorbed in their chelated form, which means that the minerals are bonded to protein molecules that transport them to the bloodstream and enhance their absorption.

Magnesium

Magnesium is one of the most critical nutrients for your cardiovascular health. This trace mineral is required by every cell and is used to manufacture more than 300 enzymes, many of which are involved in energy production. It is needed for production and use of adenosine triphosphate (ATP), your body's energy source.

One of magnesium's major jobs is to help all the muscles in your body relax (calcium, on the other hand, makes them contract). Magnesium works in conjunction with calcium to maintain normal heart rhythm by relaxing and contracting the heart muscle. Magnesium also acts as nature's calcium channel blocker. It prevents the calcium that's not absorbed into your bones from collecting in your arteries where it can build up, clog your arteries, and increase your risk of heart attack. Magnesium has the same blocking activity, without the side effects, as two commonly used calcium channel blockers: Cardizem, Tiamate, and Tiazac (diltiazem) or Verelan, Isoptin, and Calan (verapamil). Magnesium is also needed for proper calcium metabolism.

Magnesium opens up blood vessels in your heart, arms, and legs, which improves blood flow to the heart, increases beneficial HDL cholesterol, prevents blood platelets from becoming sticky and clumping together, and keeps blood pressure regulated and stable.

Apart from its important role in the healthy functioning of your heart and circulation, magnesium has natural tranquilizing properties. It is needed to produce the important neurotransmitters, serotonin and melatonin, which affect your mood and how well you sleep. Magnesium is also critical for growth, wound healing, and healthy pregnancy.

It's not surprising that magnesium deficiencies are at the root of many cardiovascular problems and conditions involving muscles and nerves. Low magnesium is commonly seen in people with high blood pressure, irregular or rapid heartbeat, and mitral valve prolapse (a disorder of the heart valves). Magnesium is also frequently low in people with heart attacks and fatal heart arrhythmia. Low levels of magnesium are often observed in the blood cells of cardiac patients in intensive care units. A review of magnesium and the heart in *The American Journal of Medicine* found that 65 percent of all patients admitted to intensive care units show low levels of magnesium.

Besides affecting the heart and circulation, low magnesium can contribute to anxiety, constipation, depression, fatigue, premenstrual mood swings, hypoglycemia, seizure disorders, migraine headaches, osteoporosis, poor wound healing, muscle cramps, and muscle pain (fibromyalgia).

Magnesium's therapeutic uses have become so critical to care and better understood that it is routinely used in most emergency rooms and in intensive care and coronary care units. One study of more than 100 heart attack victims who were emergency-room admittees found that the survival rate increased tenfold when patients were given intravenous magnesium. In another study, magnesium was used to aid recovery after coronary bypass surgery. A Boston study tracked 100 bypass patients, half of whom were given an injection of magnesium after surgery, while the other half were injected with a placebo. Sixteen percent of the magnesium group suffered heart-rhythm problems, while more than twice as many— 34 percent—of the placebo group experienced such problems.

Researchers have also found a correlation between magnesium levels and elevation in blood pressure—the lower the body's level of magnesium, the higher the blood pressure. It has also been observed that supplemental magnesium can result in significant reductions in both systolic and diastolic blood pressure that are dependent on the dose of magnesium taken. One large-scale ongoing study mentioned earlier that was begun in 1980, called the Nurses' Health Study, followed 58,218 nurses over a four-year period and through a series of questionnaires recorded their eating habits and risk of developing high blood pressure. Over 3,200 women developed high blood pressure during this time. Researchers found that age, obesity, and excess alcohol consumption were the strongest predictors, but also that the amounts of magnesium and calcium consumed were also predictors. Women whose diets provided at least 300 mg of magnesium a day and 800 mg of calcium were at significantly less risk for high blood pressure than women whose diets contained less of these minerals.

Magnesium therapy is also often used to combat a common deficiency that results when diuretics are prescribed to treat high blood pressure. It is well known that diuretics lower potassium, but they also cause more magnesium to be excreted in the urine as well. Magnesium supplements help maintain adequate potassium supplementation in diuretic therapy and Bartter's syndrome (potassium wasting).

Magnesium has been used in the treatment of hypertension in pregnancy for decades. In the last trimester of pregnancy, blood pressure can elevate to dangerous levels. Studies show that levels of magnesium, calcium, phosphorous, potassium, fiber, vegetable proteins, and vitamins C and D showed an inverse relationship with blood pressure, with magnesium's correlation being the strongest.

Two of the largest drains of magnesium from the body are diet and stress. The typical American diet tends to be low in magnesium. Animal protein, fat, sugar, alcohol and caffeine cause magnesium to be excreted in the urine. Stress hormones also have the same affect. When they get too high, it causes magnesium to spill out into the urine. Interestingly, type-A personalities (overachievers) tend to lose their magnesium more easily under stress and thus show a correlation in their tendency to develop high blood pressure and ischemic heart disease. Magnesium loss also occurs with trauma and surgery, in extreme athletic exertion, and in alcoholism.

Because of the widespread prevalence of magnesium deficiency, many of our patients receive magnesium supplements. The red blood cell test and white blood cell test are believed to be the best indicators of magnesium levels—although some studies have shown that no blood tests are accurate enough to measure deficiencies of this mineral. Even when these tests are normal, magnesium supplements above and beyond normal levels can be useful, particularly in treating high blood pressure, PMS, seizure disorders, depression, constipation, chronic fatigue, and cardiac arrhythmia.

Magnesium is abundant in most animal proteins, especially dairy products, fish, meat, and seafood. Rainbow-rich sources include apples, apricots, bananas, black beans, broccoli, brown rice, cantaloupe, chickpeas, figs, garlic, grapefruit, leafy green vegetables, lemons, lima beans, millet, nuts, peaches, salmon, sesame seeds, soybeans, tofu, and wheat and whole grains.

Calcium

Calcium is the most abundant mineral in the body. Although the majority of this mineral is used to make bone, a small, but critical, percentage is used for healthy heart and nerve function. You need calcium to help muscles contract and to promote normal blood clotting. It also plays a major role in electrical conduction and transmission of nerve impulses. Research has shown that a calcium-rich diet can help to lower your blood pressure. A deficiency of calcium is associated with elevated blood cholesterol, heart palpitations, high blood pressure, muscle cramps, and many other conditions. If sufficient amounts of calcium are not available, your body will pull calcium out of your bones. This can lead to osteoporosis or "brittle bones."

Numerous studies in the United States, such as the Nurses' Health Study, suggest that calcium plays an important role in high blood pressure. Many people with high blood pressure have diets low in calcium. A comparison of significant deficiencies in dietary calcium, potassium, magnesium, and vitamins A and C, shows that, of them all, low calcium is the most consistent dietary risk factor for high blood pressure. A study in the *New England Journal of Medicine* reported that when people with mild to moderate hypertension were given 1,000 mg of calcium a day for four months, their blood pressure was significantly lowered. It appears that calcium may lower elevated blood pressure by increasing sodium excretion.

In contrast, several studies have shown that taking too much calcium can be as much of a problem as taking too little. High blood levels of calcium in conditions such as chronic hypercalcemia (a severe increase of calcium levels in the blood), hyperthyroidism, or vitamin D toxicity, are all associated with increased chronic high blood pressure. Excessive amounts of calcium can also contribute to irregular heartbeat and heart palpitations.

Because of these findings, we use calcium sparingly except in cases where a woman patient is suspected of having osteoporosis or when blood calcium levels are normal yet additional tests such as urine telepetides, ionized calcium, or red blood cell calcium indicate a loss of calcium. Calcium can't be well absorbed without vitamin D; so when we use calcium supplements, we use them with vitamin D.

A diet that is high in protein, fat, or sugar affects calcium uptake. The average American diet of refined grains, meats, and soft drinks (all are high in phosphorus), increases the excretion of calcium. Alcohol, coffee, junk foods, excess salt, and/or white flour lead to the loss of calcium by the body.

Good Rainbow Diet calcium sources include dark green leafy vegetables—especially broccoli, kale, and spinach—almonds, oats, soybeans, tofu, sardines and salmon, and low-fat yogurt.

When supplementing with calcium, the best form for absorption is calcium oxide or calcium citrate.

Potassium

Like magnesium and calcium, potassium enables your muscles to work properly. It is important for a regular heart rhythm, but also for relaxing the smooth muscle cells that line your blood vessels. Potassium relaxes these minute muscle cells and dilates the blood vessels. Its action is similar to the blood-pressure medications known as vasodilators, only without the side effects.

Another reason potassium is important for lowering blood pressure is that it helps the body excrete sodium. Sodium, as you know, raises blood pressure. Likewise, low potassium intake may be a significant factor in the development of high blood pressure. Numerous studies have demonstrated that the balance between your potassium and sodium levels is important for lowering and maintaining healthy blood pressure. A higher ratio of potassium-to-sodium has been found to lower moderately high blood pressure. Potassium supplementation has proven useful in diuretic-induced hypokalemia (abnormally low levels of potassium).

In the DASH study (Dietary Approaches to Stop Hypertension), which we mentioned in the previous chapter, when a group of hypertensives eating the typical American diet high in fat and sodium and low in fruits and vegetables were compared to hypertensives following a diet low in fat and nearly three times higher in fruits and vegetables, blood pressure dropped significantly in the group consuming the healthier foods. Blood pressure did not drop at all in the group eating foods typical of the American diet.

Potassium supplementation has proven beneficial, not only for treating high blood pressure, but animal studies have also found potassium supplementation lessened brain hemorrhages, heart attacks, and death rate.

The typical American diet does not supply sufficient amounts of potassium. Fresh fruits and vegetables are high in potassium. Foods on the Rainbow Diet rich in potassium include acorn squash, apricots, bananas, lima beans, broccoli, brown rice, chickpeas, dates, figs, dried fruit, garlic, nuts, potatoes, raisins, spinach, winter squash, wheat bran, yams, and yogurt.

Zinc

A trace mineral, zinc is most known for its ability to help the immune system fight infections. However, this antioxidant is also important as an antidote to heavy metals toxicity. The accumulation of metals such as aluminum, cadmium, and lead in the body have been shown to elevate blood pressure and contribute to atherosclerosis. Zinc is also beneficial for protecting blood vessels by decreasing oxidation of fats that build up and damage the lining of artery walls. Research shows that the higher the intake of dietary zinc, the lower the blood pressure.

High levels of copper, both a mineral and heavy metal, can suppress zinc levels. Numerous studies have suggested that elevations in serum copper can raise blood pressure. Excess dietary copper can increase systolic blood pressure in rats. In smokers, elevations in serum copper and cadmium have been found, which may be the reason why smokers have elevated blood pressure. Contraceptive pill users have elevated levels of serum copper and elevations in arterial pressure. Users of diuretics have significantly higher serum copper levels, which are known to deplete zinc.

Serum zinc levels are significantly lower for older women with high blood pressure and older men with high systolic readings. Heart attack victims, as well as those with coronary heart disease risk factors, show significantly decreased levels of zinc.

Blood lead levels, which are elevated in alcoholics, have been correlated with increases in blood pressure. An abundance of lead can lead to a form of hypertension with renal impairment. Elevations of lead and cadmium with decreases in zinc are a factor in many people with hypertension living in inner cities, where older buildings still contain lead-based paint and lead piping for the water supply is common.

All our patients with high blood pressure receive zinc to reduce the body's burden of heavy metals. Zinc in combination with vitamin C may be an even more effective way of reducing levels of heavy metals, especially lead and cadmium.

Zinc is found in the following sources of Rainbow Diet-permitted foods: egg yolks, fish, legumes, mushrooms, oysters, pecans, poultry, pumpkin seeds, sardines, soybeans, sunflower seeds, and whole grains.

Chromium (GTF)

The body uses the trace mineral chromium (sometimes also called glucose tolerance factor or GTF) to metabolize sugar and fat. It helps insulin work more efficiently to move blood sugar (glucose) from the blood to the cells. When levels of chromium are low, glucose isn't delivered to the cells for energy but is left to circulate in the bloodstream, where it can increase free-radical formation and blood vessel inflammation. Symptoms of chromium deficiency include elevated levels of blood sugar, cholesterol, and triglycerides, and lowered levels of beneficial HDL cholesterol.

Low chromium levels can be an indication of cardiovascular disease. In studies, patients dying of atherosclerosis had significantly lower chromium concentrations in their aortas (the main artery conducting blood from the heart) than a control group of patients with coronary artery and heart diseases. Both chromium and the mineral selenium (see following section) may have a role in the nutritional control of high blood pressure, specifically in the protection from myocardial infarction during a medical crisis.

Lack of dietary chromium is widespread in America. Not only are our soils depleted of chromium, but our diets, which for most Americans tends to be excessively high in sugar and refined carbohydrates, deplete the body's chromium reserves as well. (See "Chromium Reduces Sugar Cravings" on page 95.) The few foods that are rich sources of chromium are plentiful

Chromium Reduces Sugar Cravings

Cravings for sugar and other high-carbohydrate foods often occur in people with hypoglycemia, diabetes, and depression, and also in people deficient in chromium. Refined foods deplete chromium levels in the body and raise blood sugar levels. The more sweets and refined foods you eat, the greater the chromium deficiency, which in turn perpetuates a more intense desire for sweets. Chromium supplements have been found to diminish the urge for sweets by improving the body's insulin sensitivity, thus keeping blood sugar levels more even.

Low levels of the brain chemical serotonin are also thought to trigger cravings for sugar and high-carbohydrate foods. Serotonin regulates appetite, as well as mood, emotions, and sleep. It is made from the amino acid tryptophan and tryptophan supplementations frequently decrease sugar craving. High-protein diets with a high tryptophan-to-carbohydrate ratio also reduce sugar cravings. Other supplemental remedies that can possibly help control this impulse disorder include the amino acid glutamine, the B vitamins, and the trace minerals zinc and lithium.

in the Rainbow Diet: apples, broccoli, barley, brown rice, chicken, eggs, nuts, mushrooms, rhubarb, tomatoes, and sweet potatoes.

Chromium is best absorbed when it is taken in a form called chromium picolinate (chromium chelated with picolinate, a naturally occurring amino acid metabolite).

Selenium

Selenium plays a vital role in the production of glutathione, a powerful detoxifying and antioxidant compound. Among its many protective benefits, glutathione inhibits the oxidation of fats and neutralizes toxins in the liver. A potent antioxidant itself, selenium helps to detoxify the body of mercury and other heavy metals. It aids in the production of antibodies, boosting immune function, and it can protect against the formation of some types of tumors. Selenium has been found to work in tandem with vitamin E to protect against serious viruses such as the Coxsackie virus, which can inflame the heart, causing cardiomyopathy and heart failure.

Low levels of selenium have been linked to cancer and heart disease, and are associated with high cholesterol levels. Selenium levels in patients with acute myocardial infarction were determined to be low before, and not as a result of, this condition.

Due to food processing and low mineral levels in soil, the average American diet is deficient in selenium. Good sources of selenium in the Rainbow Diet include Brazil nuts (which have the highest selenium content of any food), broccoli, brown rice, chicken, garlic, onions, salmon, vegetables, and whole grains.

AMINO ACIDS

One of the many important roles of amino acids is to provide the materials needed by the body to manufacture neurotransmitters. Medicine has focused its treatment efforts on drugs to fight the symptoms of high blood pressure and heart disease and, sadly, has missed the opportunity to transform high blood pressure and heart disease risk by treating it at one point of origin, the central nervous system. Adjustment of the patient's neurotransmitters is critical to long-term cardiovascular disease reversal. For this reason, the following amino acids are nearly always an integral part of our treatment program.

Unless otherwise noted below, we advocate use of the L-form amino aid supplements. This form of amino acid is also called free-form. This means that the amino acid supplement is already in its simplest form and is not part of a larger protein. Free-form amino acids are generally the best form for absorption throughout the body and brain.

Arginine

Arginine is a nonessential amino acid that is thought to work through its ability to manufacture nitric oxide (NO). NO is a simple molecule made up of nitrogen and oxygen. It can permeate nearly all cell membranes where it helps to regulate many functions. In the cells lining the arteries, NO regulates the tone of the endothelial cells. These cells regulate the normal dilating, or relaxing, of blood vessels necessary for normal blood flow, which in turn, helps the body maintain normal, healthy, blood pressure. If these cells become dysfunctional, the blood vessels constrict, leading to reduced blood flow or spasms, which can result in high blood pressure.

A small but impressive study from Italy found that a twofold increase in arginine substantially reduced blood pressure. In this study, participants were divided into three groups, each of which ate three different diets containing varying amounts of arginine. The first group consumed foods that resulted in a total of three to four grams of arginine a day. The second group ate arginine-rich foods equal to approximately 10 grams a day. The third group followed the same diet as the first group, and also took 10 grams of arginine in supplement form. Just one week later, significant drops in blood pressure were observed in groups two and three, but not in group one.

NO is thought to enhance circulation and performance throughout the body, including the arteries, immune system, liver, pancreas, uterus, penis, peripheral nerves, lungs, and brain. Low levels of arginine in the body compromise production of NO and a variety of other functions such as growth hormone release, insulin production, cholesterol regulation, fat metabolism by the liver, sexual function and fertility, and wound healing.

Foods on the Rainbow Diet high in arginine include carob, chocolate, coconut, fish, oats, peanuts, poultry, soybeans, walnuts, wheat and whole grains.

Carnitine

Carnitine is made in the body from the amino acids lysine and methionine. It is used within the cells to burn fat for energy production, and as such, provides a number of actions particularly important to the heart. Studies have shown that carnitine lowers total cholesterol and trigylceride levels and raises HDL cholesterol. It also lowers blood pressure in those with hypertension and improves such conditions as angina, arrthythmia, and heart failure.

Red meat and dairy products contain the greatest amounts of carnitine. The Rainbow Diet allows you to choose low-fat or fat-free dairy products and to eat lean red meat sparingly.

Note: People who are on hemodialysis should supplement with L-carnitine only under the supervision of a physician.

Methionine (or Cysteine)

Methionine is an essential amino acid that contributes to the breakdown of fats, which helps to prevent an accumulation of fat in the liver and arteries that might obstruct blood circulation to the kidneys, heart, and brain. It is also the precursor to cysteine, glutathione, and taurine, the body's most powerful antioxidants and detoxifiers. The body can make the amino acid cysteine only from methionine, whereas taurine can be made from methionine and cysteine. Glutathione is made from a combination of three amino acids, of which cysteine is the most important. Methionine, like all the sulfur amino acids (cysteine, taurine, and homocysteine), needs adequate amounts of the B vitamins pyridoxine, folic acid, and cobalamin to be properly metabolized.

As an essential amino acid, methionine cannot be made by the body and so must be obtained from foods or supplements. Methionine is most abundant in foods from animal sources such as eggs, fish, milk, and meat. Other good food sources from the Rainbow Diet include beans, garlic, lentils, onions, soybeans, and sunflower seeds.

Taurine

Taurine is an essential amino acid that is found in high concentrations in the heart muscle, white blood cells (the immune system's first line of defense), retina, and central nervous system, where its most important function is to facilitate the passage of sodium, potassium, calcium, and magnesium into and out of cells, and to electrically stabilize the cell membranes. Specifically, it helps to increase the strength of the heart muscle, spare the loss of potassium from it, and reduce the overactivity of the fibers that conduct the impulse for the heartbeat. As an important component of bile, taurine is used to digest fats and control cholesterol levels and, like all the other sulfur amino acids, it neutralizes heavy metals and helps eliminate them from the body.

Taurine has proven useful for many types of cardiovascular conditions, including arrhythmia, cardiomyopathy, cholesterol reduction, congestive heart failure, edema, mitral valve prolapse, and high blood pressure. Because deficiencies in methionine and cysteine (precursors of taurine) are widespread, most of our patients with high blood pressure or other forms of heart disease receive supplemental taurine.

Organ meats, particularly brains, are excellent food sources of taurine. However, these are not recommended foods on the Rainbow Diet. Taurine, in general, is not found in significant concentrations in food.

Tryptophan

Tryptophan is an essential amino acid that works primarily in the central nervous system where it is converted to serotonin and melatonin, both important brain chemicals that help regulate your mood, appetite, and sleep. Tryptophan is most often used to fight depression, stabilize emotions, control hyperactivity, alleviate stress, and aid in weight loss and healthy sleep patterns, which indirectly help to discourage hypertension and heart disease. Studies have also linked low levels of tryptophan to an increased risk of heart attack. In dosages of 3.5 grams a day, tryptophan has been found to lower blood pressure. Sufficient levels of tryptophan are also needed for the production of niacin, which decreases heart disease by lowering cholesterol levels.

Due to a number of deaths in 1989 caused by a contaminated batch of tryptophan, the amino acid was banned from the market. The ban was rescinded in 1996, but tryptophan is now available only by prescription.

Tryptophan is the least abundant essential amino acid in foods. It is not typically found in any significant amount in the normal diet, and most dietary proteins are deficient in this amino acid. Beef and pork contain relatively large amounts of tryptophan, as do salted anchovies, but these foods are not encouraged on the Rainbow Diet. Usable sources of tryptophan include almonds, brown rice, cottage cheese, eggs, peanuts, Parmesan and Swiss cheeses, and soy protein.

FOOD SUPPLEMENTS

A few of the nutrients in our program can be obtained in food and also in supplement form. These include garlic, pectin, fiber, and fish oils. The cardiovascular benefits of these foods were discussed in the previous chapter. We'll simply recap their benefits here and provide the information on their supplement form.

Garlic

To benefit from the antioxidant protection and cholesterol and blood pressure lowering action of garlic, you need to consume one to three fresh cloves a day. Raw garlic, cooked garlic, and garlic-infused oil all give you the benefits of garlic. For some people, this may be a challenge. As an alternative, odorless, dried garlic or aged garlic is available in tablet, capsule, or liquid form.

Fiber

Dietary fiber comes from the thick cell wall of plants. It is an indigestible complex carbohydrate. Fiber is divided into two types: water soluble and water insoluble. Besides containing an abundance of vitamins, minerals, phytochemicals, and antioxidants, most fruits (but not fruit juice), vegetables, beans, whole grains, nuts, and seeds contain lots of fiber. Fiber aids in lowering cholesterol, stabilizing blood sugar, and helps in the removal of toxins and heavy metals. Fiber can also be useful if you have constipation or colon problems such as polyps or diverticulitis.

The best way to get fiber is from food. Whole grains are particularly high in insoluble fiber. Oats, barley, beans, fruits, and vegetables contain significant amounts of both types of fiber and are the best sources of soluble fiber. Your fiber intake should be sufficient on the Rainbow Diet, however, if you don't include enough, fiber supplements are an option.

Fiber supplements come in powder and capsule form. Choose a fiber supplement that contains different types of fiber—both soluble and insoluble fiber. We don't recommend Metamucil, a common over-the-counter, bulk-forming laxative, which tends to cause flatulence in many. Citrucel (sugar-free) is a better option.

Pectin

Pectin is a form of soluble fiber that is found in the cell walls of plants and in the skins and rinds of fruits and vegetables. Pectin helps to lower LDL cholesterol and remove unwanted toxins and heavy metals from the body. Pectin is available in powder and capsule form.

The Rainbow Diet and its various nutritional supplements are two of the three most powerful tools you have for treating high blood pressure and heart disease and for keeping your heart and circulatory system healthy. The third and final part of the No-More Hypertension and Heart Disease Program, which we'll move on to now, presents several adjunct therapies and simple lifestyle changes that can have a big impact on reversing your hypertension and heart disease.

CHAPTER 6

Stress Reduction, Lifestyle Changes, and Other Healing Therapies

While the Rainbow Diet and supplement support can go a long way toward treating and protecting against high blood pressure and heart disease, for some it may not be enough. Other therapies and lifestyle factors can strongly influence the health of your heart and arteries. Exercise, weight control, stress management, and hormone and chelation therapies can also play a prominent role in helping you to achieve optimal cardiovascular health.

STRESS REDUCTION

Dealing with the stressors in your life should be a top priority. When you are stressed or feel overly anxious, these emotions stimulate the sympathetic nervous system, which in turn, floods the body with stress chemicals known as adrenaline and cortisol. These substances accelerate heart rate, blood pressure, oxygen consumption, and blood flow to the muscles. Nearly all body functions and organs respond to stress, and therefore can manifest in any number of physical symptoms, including:

- Acne
- Constipation
- Cough
- Diarrhea
- Difficulty swallowing
- Eyestrain
- Fatigue

- Frequent urination
- Gastrointestinal complaints
- Headache
- Heart palpitations
- Hyperventilation
- Insomnia

- Light-headedness
- Numbness in the hands and toes
- Painful muscle spasms
- Sweaty hands or cold hands

Stress is an unavoidable part of life. But if you regularly "fall apart," eventually it starts to depress the immune system and wear down the body. Researchers estimate that long-term stress contributes to as many as 80 percent of all major illnesses. Free-radical damage, elevated cholesterol, high blood pressure, and an increase in stroke or heart attack are a few of the effects of long-term stress on the cardiovascular system. Clearly the mind and the body are one, but in the long run using anti-anxiety drugs like Valium (diazepam), Xanax (alprazolam), or Dilantin (phenytoin) is not the best way to deal with stress. It's more important to learn how to defuse stress and to maintain a sense of mental balance. By "keeping cool" under life's daily pressures, you may avoid all these stress-related problems and be a much happier—and healthier—person.

Among the many studies to show a correlation between stress and high blood pressure, *The Journal of Hypertension* found that, interestingly, people who control their own schedule and own pace seem to feel less stress. According to the study, it is not the type of work you do, but the amount of control you feel you have over it that makes the mercury move on the stress gauge. It is wise to be able to distinguish between the stresses you can control and those you cannot. Once you do this, your opportunities to reverse high blood pressure and heart disease can improve greatly.

Modern medicine has begun to recognize that all disease is partly psychosomatic—that is, our outlook and anticipation of the future strongly influence the course of our wellness or sickness. The most effective healthcare is focused on mental and physical health together. Fortunately, the skills to address the stressors in our lives can be learned quite easily. There are a wide variety of relaxation techniques to choose from: guided imagery, biofeedback, cranial electrical stimulation (CES), meditation, or prayer. This section focuses on the relaxation techniques that we have found to be most valuable for reducing anxiety and stress. Relaxation techniques that focus on brain-wave activity have the widest benefits because the nervous system and the brain influence more body functions than any other.

Brain waves tend to create certain patterns, which scientists have classified in four types:

- Alpha waves—associated with states of deep physical relaxation and calmness during which the mind is awake but unfocused

- Beta waves—dominant during conscious activity; a state of alertness

- Delta waves—prominent during unconscious "deep" sleep and dreaming states

- Theta waves—present when the mind is drifting from a conscious to an unconscious state; a mysterious elusive state associated with access to unconscious material, intense memories, creative inspiration, and enlightened insights

Studies have shown that when the brain is emitting alpha waves, the body increases its production of endorphins (the body's natural painkillers) and stimulates the conversion of amino acids into neurotransmitters. Neurotransmitters act as chemical messengers in the body. Serotonin, for example, is a well-known neurotransmitter that is considered essential for relaxation, sleep, and concentration.

Learning to manage stress through one or more of the following mind-body techniques is one of the most helpful things you can do to protect your heart and arteries.

Cranial Electrical Stimulation

Cranial electrical stimulation (CES) is a gentle therapeutic procedure that generates minute, low-voltage electrical stimulation to the brain for the purpose of treating stress-related disorders. Also known as electrotherapy, cerebral electrical therapy (CET), or neurotonic or neuroelectrical therapy (NET), CES is thought to work by increasing alpha waves, the brain-wave activity associated with states of deep physical relaxation during which the mind is awake but unfocused. CES has been found to produce effects on the body and mind similar to those achieved by meditation.

CES has been successfully used to help with pain relief, hard-to-heal bone fractures, irregular heart rhythms, and even with stroke victims attempting to regain movement in their hands. Other potential applications for CES include relief of menstrual cramping, stiff neck, allergic reactions, headache, drug addiction, and temporal lobe disorders (typically stress and anxiety-related disorders that are caused by brain chemical imbalances). But by far their greatest success has been found in the clinical treatment of anxiety, depression, insomnia, and stress. More than 100 published studies on CES have appeared in the medical literature, documenting its effectiveness in treating these conditions:

- Anxiety: An average improvement of over 50 percent in test scores of hospitalized psychiatric patients and inpatient alcoholics with measured anxiety.

- Stress related to withdrawal syndrome in inpatient substance abusers: Reduced stress measurements, in every instance, by at least 40 percent.

- Depression: An average reduction of 50 percent in the depression scores of long-term psychiatric patients, university counseling-center clients, post-withdrawal alcoholic patients, and hospitalized para- and quadriplegics.

- Insomnia: Significant improvement in sleep onset time, sleep efficiency, percentage of bedtime sleep, and percentage of sleep time in delta, or "deep," sleep.

The use of electricity in therapeutic disorders dates back in scientific history to Anton Mesmer, who tried to use magnetism for the treatment of a variety of medical problems. Allen Childs, M.D., Assistant Professor of Pharmacy at the University of Texas at Austin, suggests that electrical therapies actually date back to ancient Egypt.

Present-day applications for CES began in Europe in the 1950s under the rubric "electrosleep." Eastern nations soon picked it up as a treatment modality, and by the late 1960s its use had spread worldwide. During this time, animal studies of CES began in the United States at the University of Tennessee and at what is now the University of Wisconsin Medical School. These were soon followed by human clinical trials at the University of Texas Medical School in San Antonio, the University of Mississippi Student Counseling Center, and the University of Wisconsin Medical School. By the early 1970s, the Food and Drug Administration (FDA) had approved CES devices for clinical treatment of anxiety, depression, insomnia, and stress, and even drug abuse, in which anxiety and depression frequently play a part.

CES is performed by placing simple, non-irritating electrodes on the forehead and on the left inner wrist over the pulse. These, in turn, are attached by wires to a transcutaneous electric nerve stimulation (TENS) unit, a small monitor that can be attached to a belt at your waist. Minute, gentle electric signals are then sent to the vagus nerve in the brain, which stimulates the release of two critical amino acids gamma-butyric acid (GABA) and acetylcholine. In the brain, GABA functions as an inhibitory neurotransmitter, decreasing neuron activity and nerve cells from over-firing, which has a calming, relaxing effect. Acetylcholine, on the other hand, is a stimulating neurotransmitter and enhances the ability of brain cells to communicate with one another, which helps the brain's speed, memory, and ability to think clearly.

Treatment with CES is typically fifteen, thirty, or sixty minutes twice a day for stress; depending on physician and treatment goals (this may vary). Some individuals with severe addictions may require four to eight hours of treatment a day. People often report experiencing a benefit in the first thirty-minute session. CES therapy may initially produce a tingling sensation—a positive and normal reaction. Another marker of its benefits is that it will produce a deep sense of relaxation and even improve sleep. For other individuals, an appropriate trial period, in which CES is used concurrently with amino acids or antidepressants, may be necessary. The therapy can require at least three weeks, and sometimes as much as two months, to reach its full benefit.

CES therapy is safe, noninvasive, nonaddictive, and has no known pharmaceutical side effects. It is contraindicated in epileptics, women who are pregnant, or people who have pacemakers. Treatment must be prescribed and monitored by a health professional, but may be performed at home. Several thousand Americans are treated with CES annually and more than 11,000 people own CES devices.

We live in a technological age, surrounded by electromagnetic fields and currents, and that electromagnetic "pollution" generated from our video screens, televisions, stereophonic equipment, microwaves and phone lines may actually be impacting our health. Electromagnetic fields cause brain waves to go from alpha to theta and lose their basic relaxing state. CES may provide natural levels of supplementary current to keep the brain healthy. Thus, CES treatment may prove to be a necessary antidote, not only for reversing hypertension and heart disease, but also for maintaining fully optimum health.

Biofeedback-Training Techniques

Biofeedback attempts to connect the mind to the body. It is a form of self-awareness training that combines a variety of relaxation techniques with the use of equipment. The combination enables you to become more aware of the effects of your emotions on body functions. Over time, with the help of a well-trained biofeedback therapist, you can learn to consciously regulate a number of your own involuntary or autonomic nervous system functions, including respiration, heart rate, blood pressure, pulse, skin temperature, and brain-wave activity that were once thought to be beyond your conscious control, and that contribute to high blood pressure and heart disease.

Until recently it was thought that unconscious, involuntary processes formally sent feedback signals only to the hypothalamus. The hypothalamus serves as the primary link between the nervous system and the endocrine glands. The hypothalamus senses conditions from the environment such as temperature, light, and even emotional feelings, and relays this information to the pituitary, which in turn regulates the amount of hormone production among several endocrine glands. We have now learned how to activate regions of the left and right prefrontal cortex—an area of the brain just behind the forehead that recent research has associated with positive emotion (the left side) and anxiety, depression, and other mood disorders (the right side). This allows us to bridge the normal gap between conscious and unconscious, and voluntary and involuntary, processes. With biofeedback, people can learn to recognize essential stress cues they might not normally recognize. Helping individuals to understand the connection between body and mind and how their mind and emotions impact their heart rate, temperature, vascular system, pulse rate, bowel and bladder, and other functions, is the first step we teach in biofeedback.

During a typical biofeedback therapy session, electrodes are taped to the skin and connected to a monitor, which can track any number of physiological responses. As you practice a relaxation technique, the monitor uses sounds, images, or flashes of light to give you feedback about how effective you are in reaching your desired effect. For example, if you are trying to relax your muscles, variations in sound can indicate your degree of relaxation, moment by moment. If your aim is to slow your pulse, sounds or lights make your pulse more tangible than by just feeling the pulse. By hearing or seeing the pulse, it is easier to try to manipulate or control it consciously. If you are a cardiac patient with premature contractions (a common type of irregular heartbeat induced by anxiety), you can learn to stabilize it by listening to your own heartbeat on a loudspeaker, and following it as you relax. By giving auditory and/or visual signals, individuals are able to better direct their conscious thoughts and thus control what would normally be outside their control.

Biofeedback training has already proven effective in treating a wide range of conditions associated with stress and anxiety. These conditions include high blood pressure, irregular heartbeat, palpitations, agoraphobia, asthma, cerebral palsy, certain forms of poor circulation such as Raynaud's disease, chronic anxiety, depression, headaches (migraine and tension), epilepsy, impotence, peptic ulcer, colitis, irritable bowel syndrome, hyperactivity, learning disabilities, muscle spasm, PMS (premenstrual syndrome), psychiatric conditions, substance abuse disorders, smoking, sleep disorders, and tinnitus.

Many muscular-skeletal problems such as prolonged immobilization, joint repair, muscle tendon transfer, whiplash, and muscle shortening also respond to biofeedback treatment.

When biofeedback is combined with CES, it becomes a powerful tool for deflecting negative emotions such as anger, hostility, frustration, and depression, all of which contribute to heart disease. (See "Negative Emotions and Personality Types" on page 116.)

With continued practice of the relaxation exercises and the opportunity to hear or watch the body's responses, you can eventually learn to provoke the desired response using the relaxation technique, but without the use of the machine. This mastery can then be called upon to help provide support whenever it is needed, and to achieve a level of self-control and peace of mind you may not have thought possible.

Alpha Brain-Wave Training

Alpha brain-wave training is a particularly useful form of biofeedback because the brain has no sensory processes by which it can detect its own type of brain-wave activity. Your hands may feel cold, but you may not know that theta-wave activity (a drowsy, dreamlike state that occurs when the mind is drifting from a conscious to an unconscious state) is dominating the brain rather than alpha-wave activity, which occurs when you are awake and relaxed. You can get a sense of the brain's control through this technique of biofeedback. One of the primary goals of alpha-feedback training is to increase alpha waves (which normally decrease with age), thereby bringing both alpha and theta waves into balance.

Alpha feedback training relies on the use of sound to increase alpha brain-wave activity. The lower limit of our ability to hear is 25 hertz, but the average alpha frequency is only 10 hertz, which is inaudible without amplification. By multiplying the alpha frequency by 200, the average alpha feedback tone then lies within the range of the human hearing spectrum and generates a series of musical tones which can sound like flute music. In contrast, theta feedback sounds more like an oboe. A sound monitor, which is attached to electrodes, is placed on the head and the frequency of the flutelike tone indicates when alpha brain-wave activity is greater than 40 percent of the time. When alpha activity reaches 50 percent, theta training can replace alpha, if it too is low. When theta percent reaches 50 percent, biofeedback for both alpha and theta feedback can be balanced and maintained with a different bell for each.

Augmenting alpha and theta brain waves in order to bring them into balance can also help individuals reduce anxiety and all its emotional and physical manifestations, such as headaches, irritable bowel syndrome, overeating, stomach problems, heart palpitations, ulcers, and other brain chemically mediated stress conditions such as arthritis, memory loss, and back pain.

Guided imagery, which you will read about next, can also help equalize alpha and theta waves.

Guided Imagery

A form of biofeedback known as guided imagery is the envisioning of images or scenes in order to bring about a positive physical change. There is a substantial body of research documenting the effects of positive thoughts and emotions to stimulate immune function, reduce stress, slow heartbeat, and more. In treatment, guided imagery has been used successfully in the reversal of stress that leads to heart disease, as well as in the treatment of rheumatoid arthritis, cancer, and other illnesses.

We have found an effective method for helping our patients zero in on images that work best for them. We ask a patient to start by imagining a

Biofeedback and Spirituality

Self-regulation is at the core of biofeedback, but many people believe that regulation by a higher power is ultimately what is accomplished. Those who wish to approach biofeedback from a religious perspective may apply the following suggestions to achieve similar benefits:

• The use of imagery in biofeedback can be selected from prophetic images, for example: God and His chariot (Ezekiel); the scroll extended from heaven to earth (Revelation); turning water into wine (John); walking on water (Gospels); the dead coming back to life (Revelation). By using prophetic imagery in the context of biofeedback, one can maximize the healing effect of imagery on the brain's physical nervous system.

• The use of a form of biofeedback that emphasizes meditative quiet. The Biblical principle here is "Be still and know that the Lord is God." There is a time during which a person must be still in order to experience his/her connection to a higher power.

• The use of an aspect of biofeedback that works on repetitive thought processing and cognitive drilling. This is equivalent to repetitive or contemplative prayer, which can be used during the biofeedback process to increase the alpha-theta transition state.

series of peaceful images linked to important facets of his or her life. They include peaceful images related to family, the world, finance, self, work, and community or society. Afterward, the patient numbers these images in order of importance and chooses three or four to focus upon in their ongoing work. If you choose to use guided imagery during biofeedback, work with your doctor or healthcare practitioner to develop the mental pictures that work best for you.

Meditation

For decades scientific research has known that meditation reduces physical markers of stress such as heart rate, perspiration, and blood pressure. Much of this research on the health benefits of meditation has been done on transcendental meditation (TM). TM involves repeating a word or mantra to calm the mind and keep it focused on the present. The other two most common types of meditation are mindfulness meditation, which

---

• The use of still another form of biofeedback—relaxing and experiencing the Sabbath peace. The practice of biofeedback can improve one's ability to willfully relax and therefore makes it easier to "turn off" one day per week in a society that never turns off and never stops. Relaxation training, therefore, can be an important part of the Biblical path.

• The use of biofeedback to help an individual learn to control the vascular and nervous system in his or her body. The Biblical principle here is that the brain controls the body as the heavens control the earth, therefore, the heart and pulse rate and other bodily functions can be controlled by the brain. Biofeedback can be viewed as a way of extending the heavenly and spiritual control of the brain into the body.

• Scientists claim that by using biofeedback you can gain answers to your problems from listening to your inner self. Believers in God know that the Kingdom of God is within them—the source of all truth. This connection to God, or Higher Consciousness, can be achieved by increasing the alpha state. God has given us the spirit of self-control and any technique that helps us master self-control is moving us along the path toward total holiness. By reading and meditating on God's "Word" in conjunction with special biofeedback techniques, one can reach a higher state of consciousness or Godliness.

involves sitting quietly and disengaging from external events and emotions without reacting to them, and breath meditation, which concentrates the attention using slow, deep breaths.

Biofeedback is not unlike meditation. During biofeedback the mind becomes tranquil and focused, bringing about a sense of deep relaxation, quiet, and inner calm. It can also be used as a tool for releasing potential stress and promoting a state of physical and mental balance.

Not surprisingly, many people who use biofeedback find they are brought in touch with their own "inner path." Here in the West, we refer to this concept in many different ways: We might call this the source of each person's talent and strength, or perhaps the root of their creativity. It is sometimes called the ego, which can be defined as the transpersonal spiritual self of every person. This ego is distinct from the ego of psychology and psychiatry—it is an extension of the personality and frequently called "the soul." In China, this source of the soul is called "the Tao," or the path. In Zen it is called the "true self"; in India, "Jiva." In Sanskrit, the path is called "Antakarana." The path concept is common both in Christianity and Judaism. In the Book of Acts, early Christians were called to be "on the path." Derech HaShem, or "the path to God," has been the great tradition in Judaism.

Biofeedback shows us that there is a way to control the soul or self, as well as the body. Achieving a state of inner contentment and of knowing that you are doing what is right for you can have a profound effect not only on your mental states, but also on the physical states that contribute to high blood pressure and heart disease.

LIFESTYLE CHANGES

The primary factors that contribute to heart disease are lifestyle-related and are factors over which you have control. Apart from diet, other major lifestyle factors—include inactivity, obesity, negative emotions, and harmful habits such as smoking, and excessive alcohol consumption. Lifestyle changes are an important way to keep your heart and circulatory system healthy.

Exercise

The heart is the most active muscle in the body and, like any other muscle, it needs exercise to keep fit. Exercise increases circulation, improves insulin sensitivity, can lower blood pressure 10 to 15 points, and reduces cholesterol and triglycerides while raising HDL cholesterol. It is a great reliever of stress, depression, anxiety, and insomnia. It also increases metabolic rate, promotes weight loss, improves muscle tone, strengthens bones, increases growth hormone secretion, enhances sexual performance, and improves the body's ability to absorb and use nutrients. The benefits of exercise are limitless. Engaging in exercise will not only help you to be healthier, but also to live longer. Next to weight, exercise is the best predictor of a long lifespan.

The amount and type of exercise you should do depends on several factors including your age, health, and physical condition. Be sure to check with your physician or healthcare practitioner before starting a new exercise program. A well-rounded program should include the following forms of exercise:

- Aerobic or endurance exercise increases delivery of oxygen throughout the body and enhances blood supply to the muscles. Brisk walking, bike riding, dancing, cross-country skiing, jogging, and swimming are examples of aerobic activity.

- Weight-, strength-, or resistance-training, also a form of aerobic exercise, helps to build muscle and strength, and promotes production of growth hormone. Workouts involve the use of machines, weights, or the body to provide resistance.

- Anaerobic, or flexibility, exercise improves range-of-movement and extension in the joints and muscles. Stretching exercises such as yoga, Pilates, and Qi-gong and t'ai chi (ancient types of exercise that concentrate on movement and breath) are examples of anaerobic exercise.

When devising an exercise routine, focus first on optimizing circulation and then on relaxing the body. Exercising in this order enhances the process of protein synthesis and fat release. Any type of weight-, strength-, or resistance-training is fueled by glycogen (the main form of stored glucose) in muscle tissues, and if followed by aerobic movement, depletes glycogen stores, resulting in hormonal shifts, which amplify the release of fat. Strength-, weight-, or resistance-training exercise also increases growth hormone production, which actually takes place afterward when the body is in a state of relaxation. Do not train with weights after an intense aerobic workout or train beyond your body's ability to adequately recuperate. If you do, you reduce growth hormone production and increase production of the stress hormone cortisol, which may break down muscle tissue.

To reap the greatest exercise benefits, aim for thirty to forty-five minutes of physical activity, approximately five to six times a week. Devote half of your exercise routine to an aerobic type of exercise and the other half to anaerobic movements. Together they will optimize blood flow and strengthen not only the muscular system, but also the heart.

Keep in mind that becoming active is a gradual process. If you are not used to exercising regularly, or if you have any medical or orthopedic problems, you will need to work up to this level of exercise gradually. An excellent introduction to exercise is to begin slowly with a program of walking. Walking is a safe, effective exercise that everyone can do. Make a point to walk during your day. Walk to and from work, if possible. If that is not possible, try and park several blocks away and walk. Take the stairs instead of an elevator or escalator. Set small goals for exercise each week. For example, you may wish to begin with ten to fifteen minutes of walking, three days a week, and as you feel stronger, work your way up to thirty minutes a day, five to six days a week. Eventually you can add some weight-, strength-, or resistance-training exercise to build muscle and strength in your arms, shoulders, chest, and back. It is important to exercise consistently and moderately. Listen to your body and don't push yourself.

In general, we do not recommend endurance training. Prolonged strenuous activity increases the body's need for B vitamins, zinc, chromium, beta-carotene, and choline. Sweating heavily depletes potassium and magnesium and, if done long-term, can create heart rhythm problems, and in cases of severe depletion, death. High-intensity sport activities such as long-distance running decrease fertility and sex drive, and can also cause anemia. Although high-intensity exercise does increase endorphins, the body's natural painkillers (resulting in a runner's "high"), the overall effects of extreme exercise are not beneficial.

Weight Loss

Being overweight is a major contributing cause of high blood pressure and heart disease—as well as many other serious and preventable illnesses. Obesity is an epidemic in America, affecting 25 to 50 percent of all Americans. Carrying extra weight puts undue stress on the heart and many other body parts and organs. Getting your weight under control is crucial to bringing your blood pressure down.

The best way to determine whether you are overweight is to calculate your body mass index (BMI). BMI compares how much you weigh to how tall you are. Calculate your BMI using the table on page 114. Find your height in inches in the left column. Scan across to find your weight in pounds. Your BMI is indicated at the top of that column.

- If your BMI is less than 19, you are considered underweight.

- If your BMI is 19–24.9, you are considered a healthy, normal weight.

- If your BMI is 25–29.9, you are considered overweight.

- If your BMI is more than 30, you are considered obese.

We won't go into detail here about diets and how to lose weight. Permanent weight loss requires a lifetime commitment to a healthier eating lifestyle, as well as healthy exercise. In short, the best way to reduce weight is to eat a nutritious diet that is high in fruits, vegetables and spices, moderate in whole grains and protein, and low in fat and sweets, and to get at least thirty to forty-five minutes of exercise five to six days of the week. Although exercise won't cut your appetite, it can help to control it. Simple exercise such as walking or swimming can add years to one's life. In a study where energy expenditure per week approached 3,500 calories, illness also decreased significantly. Keeping a food diary has been shown to help people lose weight more successfully and is strongly recommended. Also, don't focus on losing pounds only. Many individuals who appear to still be overweight while dieting will actually have added muscle and lost fat. The scale cannot discern this type of information. A dual energy x-ray absorptiometry scan (DEXA scan) can determine whether or not an individual is redistributing, that is, adding muscle and losing fat. (See page 137 for more information on DEXA scans.)

Most people with excess pounds who follow the Rainbow Diet will lose weight naturally as their systems resume their normal functioning and become balanced again in response to the therapeutic nutrients and the special foods of the diet. If you are unable to lose weight after several weeks on the diet, chances are the root of the problem lies not with your metabolism, but in your brain.

Researchers are finding that obesity that is unresponsive to changes in diet can be treated through brain-chemistry manipulation. Studies examining the role of a hormone called leptin in brain development and obesity are finding that your natural appetite and weight level may originate in your brain chemistry just after birth, and may then be set for the rest of your life. This means that the amount of leptin in your body in those first few weeks of life is controlled by genetics, not by what you are fed. Leptin is secreted by the fat tissue in your body and regulates appetite. The more leptin present in your body, the less hungry you are. Researchers discovered this by experimenting with mice genetically engineered not to pro-

Body Mass Index Table

Body Weight (pounds)

Height (inches)	Normal						Overweight					Obese										Extreme Obesity															
BMI	19	20	21	22	23	24	25	26	27	28	29	30	31	32	33	34	35	36	37	38	39	40	41	42	43	44	45	46	47	48	49	50	51	52	53	54
58	91	96	100	105	110	115	119	124	129	134	138	143	148	153	158	162	167	172	177	181	186	191	196	201	205	210	215	220	224	229	234	239	244	248	253	258
59	94	99	104	109	114	119	124	128	133	138	143	148	153	158	163	168	173	178	183	188	193	198	203	208	212	217	222	227	232	237	242	247	252	257	262	267
60	97	102	107	112	118	123	128	133	138	143	148	153	158	163	168	174	179	184	189	194	199	204	209	215	220	225	230	235	240	245	250	255	261	266	271	276
61	100	106	111	116	122	127	132	137	143	148	153	158	164	169	174	180	185	190	195	201	206	211	217	222	227	232	238	243	248	254	259	264	269	275	280	285
62	104	109	115	120	126	131	136	142	147	153	158	164	169	175	180	186	191	196	202	207	213	218	224	229	235	240	246	251	256	262	267	273	278	284	289	295
63	107	113	118	124	130	135	141	146	152	158	163	169	175	180	186	191	197	203	208	214	220	225	231	237	242	248	254	259	265	270	278	282	287	293	299	304
64	110	116	122	128	134	140	145	151	157	163	169	174	180	186	192	197	204	209	215	221	227	232	238	244	250	256	262	267	273	279	285	291	296	302	308	314
65	114	120	126	132	138	144	150	156	162	168	174	180	186	192	198	204	210	216	222	228	234	240	246	252	258	264	270	276	282	288	294	300	306	312	318	324
66	118	124	130	136	142	148	155	161	167	173	179	186	192	198	204	210	216	223	229	235	241	247	253	260	266	272	278	284	291	297	303	309	315	322	328	334
67	121	127	134	140	146	153	159	166	172	178	185	191	198	204	211	217	223	230	236	242	249	255	261	268	274	280	287	293	299	306	312	319	325	331	338	344
68	125	131	138	144	151	158	164	171	177	184	190	197	203	210	216	223	230	236	243	249	256	262	269	276	282	289	295	302	308	315	322	328	335	341	348	354
69	128	135	142	149	155	162	169	176	182	189	196	203	209	216	223	230	236	243	250	257	263	270	277	284	291	297	304	311	318	324	331	338	345	351	358	365
70	132	139	146	153	160	167	174	181	188	195	202	209	216	222	229	236	243	250	257	264	271	278	285	292	299	306	313	320	327	334	341	348	355	362	369	376
71	136	143	150	157	165	172	179	186	193	200	208	215	222	229	236	243	250	257	265	272	279	286	293	301	308	315	322	329	338	343	351	358	365	372	379	386
72	140	147	154	162	169	177	184	191	199	206	213	221	228	235	242	250	258	265	272	279	287	294	302	309	316	324	331	338	346	353	361	368	375	383	390	397
73	144	151	159	166	174	182	189	197	204	212	219	227	235	242	250	257	265	272	280	288	295	302	310	318	325	333	340	348	355	363	371	378	386	393	401	408
74	148	155	163	171	179	186	194	202	210	218	225	233	241	249	256	264	272	280	287	295	303	311	319	326	334	342	350	358	365	373	381	389	396	404	412	420
75	152	160	168	176	184	192	200	208	216	224	232	240	248	256	264	272	279	287	295	303	311	319	327	335	343	351	359	367	375	383	391	399	407	415	423	431
76	156	164	172	180	189	197	205	213	221	230	238	246	254	263	271	279	287	295	304	312	320	328	336	344	353	361	369	377	385	394	402	410	418	426	435	443

Source: Adapted from the National Institutes of Health/National Heart, Lung, and Blood Institute. "Clinical Guidelines on the Identification, Evaluation, and Treatment of Overweight and Obesity in Adults: The Evidence Report." Bethesda, MD: NIH, 1998.

duce this hormone. When genetically engineered mice were left untreated, their lack of leptin made them grow fat as adults. But when given leptin in the first few weeks of life, the growing mice ate much less. Many natural treatments, hormone therapy, and such drugs as Prozac (fluoxetine), Wellbutrin (bupropion), or Nardil (phenelzine) mimic leptin's appetite-reducing properties.

Researchers are also discovering that individuals with weight-resistant obesity tend to have brain waves associated with the brain waves of addiction. The brain waves of people with addictions are frequently characterized by abnormal rhythms due to an imbalance or deficiency in one or more of the brains's major neurotransmitters: acetylcholine, dopamine, gamma-aminobutyric acid (GABA), and serotonin. These abnormal brain waves can be detected using an assessment technique—akin to a cardiogram of the brain—called brain electrical activity mapping (BEAM). BEAM analysis measures the speed and strength of neurotransmissions, metabolism, and electrical activity within the brain. This laptop-sized computerized device uses an electroencephalograph (EEG) instrument, in conjunction with auditory and visual stimuli, to evoke reactions from the brain. If abnormal brain waves are identified, nutritional supplementation, drugs when appropriate (frequently prescribed for severely overweight individuals), biofeedback training techniques, and adjustments in the intake of carbohydrates (the food to which most overweight people are addicted) can be used to alter the brain-wave patterns. Given that most obesity is the result of carbohydrate addiction, and given that addictions are destructive, repetitive behaviors that can be replaced by constructive, repetitive behaviors, the brain is the area in which the battle for weight control can ultimately be won for many people.

Breaking Addictive Habits

Learning to break addictive patterns is critical if you are to restore and maintain your good health. Addiction is not just limited to dangerous and illegal drugs such as heroin, LSD, crack or other forms of cocaine, and amphetamines. It can occur with legal substances such as alcohol, cigarettes, caffeine, and even with what are considered far less harmful substances such as carbohydrates, sugar, fat, or junk food. Addiction can also be at work in people who are in codependent or addictive relationships. Addiction, by our definition, is any behavior that a person does repetitively which they know is dangerous, destructive or unhealthy, but for a variety of reasons are unable, through will power alone, to stop.

Addiction is a factor in the development of hypertension and heart disease, as well as most chronic age-related diseases such as Alzheimer's, diabetes, and cancer. For example, strong drugs, from LSD to heroin, all cause brain damage. Cigarette smoking puts you at three times greater risk of stroke and twice the risk for heart attack and lung cancer; it is also the largest known risk factor for developing Alzheimer's disease as it constricts blood vessels and inhibits circulation. Excess consumption of alcohol dilates skin blood vessels, raises blood pressure by increasing plasma catecholamines, enlarges the heart, and increases the risk of liver, colon, and breast cancer. Caffeine is proven to elevate blood pressure and to cause pancreatic cancer. Uncontrollable eating contributes to weight gain, elevated insulin, and high blood pressure, which in turn, leads to cancer, diabetes, and cardiovascular diseases. Virtually all the major killers in our society are linked in some way to repetitive, destructive, addictive behavior.

All of us in the field of preventive medicine encourage our patients to increase their fiber intake, stop smoking, give up caffeine and alcohol, give up refined sugars and carbohydrates, avoid fried foods and salty foods, exercise regularly, have positive and productive relationships with loved ones, and get appropriate amounts of rest. All are essentially behaviors that can transform an unhealthy lifestyle into an emotionally, spiritually, and physically healthy lifestyle. But once acquired, habits can be brutal to break.

Most people who try to eat healthfully fall off the wagon relatively quickly and return to their old habits. This is because addictions are a combination of many factors involving genetics and psychosocial and environmental influences, but most important brain chemical imbalances, which show up in abnormal brain waves. As with cases of treatment-resistant obesity, the technique we have found for helping people to break their addictive cycles and reestablish healthy habits is to do a brain assessment using the BEAM analysis. This allows us to identify whether there is a biochemical imbalance or deficiency among the brain's major neurotransmitters. Following that, we recommend a course of action using natural therapeutics, hormone treatments, diet and lifestyle changes to break the addictive cycle.

Negative Emotions and Personality Types

As mentioned earlier, it is well established that negative emotions such as anger, hostility, frustration, and depression (often defined as anger turned inward) register their effect on the cardiovascular system. They are known to contribute to blockages in the large vessels supplying blood to the brain, the carotids, and likely impact other blood vessels throughout the body; they raise cholesterol and blood pressure, and subject the heart to needless stressful arousal, all of which seriously increase the risk of a fatal heart attack or stroke.

Like stress, these feelings are a natural part of life. It is when they become habitual, or ingrained in one's personality, that they become psychologically and physically destructive. The type-A personality is a good example of this. The type-A personality characterizes someone who is a perfectionist, driven, compulsive, overly controlling of one's self and others, and responding outwardly to internal pressures with impatience, hostility, and blame. Someone with a type-A personality is at increased risk of developing high blood pressure and heart disease.

Other personality types or dominant personality traits can also indicate trouble. People who are extremely antisocial or who are overly aggressive, suspicious and paranoid, attention-seeking, compulsive, or hypersensitive are a few examples of other potential candidates. Personality disorders typically result from biochemical deficiencies in one of the brain's four lobes. Most all of our cardiac patients undergo a personality indicator that we call a "Millon Personality Trait Stress Test." This allows us to identify any unhealthy personality traits, which could be contributing to their emotional and stress levels and, as such, their disease states. By adjusting an individual's brain chemistry, along with the use of diet and lifestyle modifications and biofeedback exercises, negative feelings and destructive emotions can be defused and properly channeled.

OTHER HEALING THERAPIES

If an individual's high blood pressure or heart disease is resistant to our program, more aggressive measures may need to be taken. Chelation therapy and hormone replacement therapy are two approaches that may warrant consideration.

Chelation Therapy

Chelation therapy is a safe, intravenous treatment used to rid the body of excess toxic metals and minerals. Heavy toxic metals such as cadmium, lead, and mercury are absorbed into the body, primarily through food and water. These metals are known to raise cholesterol—which eventually collects on artery walls in the form of plaque—and disrupt the functioning of other minerals in the body.

The word chelation is derived from the Greek word "chel," meaning "to claw." Chelation is a common reaction in both the biological and chemical world. The chelating agent EDTA, ethylene diamine tetra acetic acid (an amino acid), was first synthesized by the German chemist Franz Munz and used in textile and fabric production. It was originally used orally in medicine for treating lead poisoning. However, this practice tended to increase lead and heavy metal absorption from the lower intestines. Today, this method of delivery is strongly discouraged in favor of intravenous chelation.

EDTA chelation has been found to substantially reduce atherosclerosis. EDTA works by binding with excess heavy metals and calcium, which it then eliminates via the kidneys and urine. Calcium, as you may remember, is an ingredient that is intimately associated with the calcification, or formation and hardening of plaque on the artery walls. EDTA breaks up plaque, unclogs arteries, and improves blood flow throughout the body. It stabilizes the intracellular membranes of the arteries. In addition, it helps to correct enzyme inhibition, which is concomitant with the advancement of atherosclerosis. It also assists in stabilizing the electric charge of platelets, thus reducing platelet leukocyte interaction (the white blood cells that attack foreign substances), leading to a reduction in unnecessary clotting. And it can act as a calcium channel blocker to lower unnecessary constrictions in the arteries.

Although chelation therapy is used chiefly in the treatment of atherosclerosis and other circulatory disorders, it has also been effective with memory loss, senility, Alzheimer's disease, diabetic gangrene, impaired vision, kidney stones, and a host of other maladies. Certain eye diseases, for example macular degeneration where circulation is diminished, are greatly helped by EDTA chelation therapy due to its cleansing effect on the blood vessels. (See Chapter 9 for profiles of patients who have used chelation to assist in reversing cardiovascular problems.) We use an assessment tool called the Doppler Test (discussed on page 140) to help us identify the severity of an individual's vascular blockages and to determine who will best benefit from chelation therapy.

The medical application of chelation therapy has continued to grow over the last several decades, yet its practice remains controversial. This is largely due to early studies showing that EDTA removes heavy metals, as well as important nutrients from the body, especially calcium. This side effect has been severely criticized by traditional medicine. Orthodox physicians also point out that chelation robs the body of vitamins, mainly vitamin

B$_6$ (pyridoxine), and may even chelate an abundance of calcium from the bones and teeth. Newer applications of this therapy are now accompanied by a vitamin regimen designed to replace whatever is lost. The decalcification of teeth or bones, a possible side effect with chelation therapy, cannot occur when this vitamin regimen is used. These and other protocols instituted by the American Board of Chelation Therapy have reduced chelation's side effects to virtually zero.

The potential benefits of chelation therapy are currently unobtainable anywhere in orthodox medicine. It has saved countless cardiovascular patients from the horrors of bypass surgery, carotid endarterectomy, and other high-risk, low-success-rate techniques. When used in conjunction with diet and supplements, and administered by a qualified physician, it remains the best process that we know of for reversing vascular blockages. To date, more than 3 million chelation treatments have been given to over 300,000 patients. Lead, cadmium, arsenic, aluminum, and excess iron pour out of the "rusting," aged patient who undergoes chelation, resulting in a dramatic reduction of atherosclerosis and an overall feeling of increased well-being and health.

Hormone Therapy

Hormones are produced by endocrine glands such as the testicles, ovaries, adrenal glands, thyroid, and pancreas. They are powerful messenger-like substances that interact with all the major systems of the body—the cardiovascular system, the gastrointestinal system, the central nervous system, and others—to regulate every aspect of the body's function, from metabolism to temperature to sex drive. It's not surprising then that because most hormone production declines with age, the functioning of these systems subsequently declines as well. As a result, the body becomes vulnerable to various age-related conditions among them, cardiovascular disease.

Research suggests that hormone replacement therapy can have many benefits as you age. The following hormones are thought to play the greatest role in slowing the aging process and are ones we use, when needed, specifically for lowering blood pressure and stabilizing heart disease. All natural hormone therapies have been shown to positively impact heart disease. The degree of reversal and stabilization depends on each person's deficiencies, supplement level, and biochemical individuality. Because of their strong effect on the body, most hormones are available by prescription only.

Dehydroepiandrosterone (DHEA)

DHEA is the most abundant hormone in the bloodstream. It is produced primarily by the adrenal glands and serves as the precursor for many adrenal hormones, including the stress hormone cortisol, and the sex hormones estrogen, progesterone, and testosterone. For this reason, it is often called "the mother of all hormones."

Research has shown that DHEA increases lifespan, decreases body fat, and is associated with a lower incidence of heart disease, cancer, diabetes, and other age-related conditions. It has also been found to enhance the activity of the immune system, improve sleep, increase energy, and help to promote a greater sense of well-being—all important factors for supporting healthy blood pressure.

Additionally, DHEA may have an important role in cognitive enhancement. DHEA protects brain cells from Alzheimer's disease and other degenerative conditions. Brain tissues naturally contain 6.5 times more DHEA than is found in other tissues. People with Alzheimer's disease may have 48 percent less DHEA than matched controls of the same age. As such, nerve degeneration may occur readily under low DHEA conditions. Research has shown that adding low concentrations of DHEA to nerve-cell tissue cultures increases the number of neurons and their ability to establish contact.

Your levels of DHEA peak in your twenties and continue to drop naturally as you age. Stress, high insulin levels, obesity, and low levels of growth hormone also suppress DHEA production. Declining levels of DHEA are known to result in a variety of problems such as depression, declining memory, sexual dysfunction, premature aging, and the inability to handle stress.

Because of DHEA's pivotal role in the body, we test all our male and female patients between the ages fifty and seventy for their DHEA blood levels. DHEA supplements are available in natural food stores, and by prescription for larger doses.

Estrogen

Estrogen is primarily thought of as a women's sex hormone, although men also secrete small amounts. Regulated by the pituitary gland, estrogen production by the ovaries begins at the onset of menstruation and drops sharply after menopause. In addition to estrogen's role in reproduction, many non-reproductive organs and systems also require this hormone. Normal cell function in the vagina, bladder, breasts, skin, bones, arteries, heart, liver, and brain require estrogen. The decrease in estrogen that occurs at menopause increases the likelihood of heart disease, osteoporosis,

Sex and a Healthy Heart

Aging, alcohol consumption, chronic illness, diabetes, medications, high blood pressure, injury, and smoking can negatively impact the ability to have an erection. However, many cases of impotence are actually related to cardiovascular disease. One study reviewed in *Science News* showed that 39 percent of men with heart disease and 15 percent of men with hypertension were impotent. Just as with the blood vessels of the heart, the blood vessels of the penis can become damaged and narrowed from a buildup of arterial plaque. So anything that improves circulation—fish oils, niacin, and vitamin E, for example—may improve potency. Many plant-based traditional treatments using herbs such as yohimbine have been explored for their effectiveness in treating sexual dysfunction. The pharmaceutical version Yocon (yohimbine hydrochloride) increases sex drive, but be careful. In high doses (greater than 40 milligrams a day), it can drastically increase your sex drive—but also boost your blood pressure.

and colorectal cancer, as well as some unpleasant side effects such as skin atrophy, depression, hot flashes, and vaginal dryness.

The conventional medical approach to menopause is hormone replacement therapy (HRT), which typically includes the use of synthetic estrogen and progesterone. HRT is not ideal, however, and poses certain risks. HRT has been shown to increase the risk of blood clots, breast cancer, gallbladder disease, and high blood pressure. In contrast, natural hormones are hormones whose molecular structures closely resemble those of the hormones made by the body and are considered safe. The ideal hormone replacement for women is a combination of estradiol (the dominant estrogen produced by the ovaries), progesterone, and testosterone. Testosterone therapy has been found to be beneficial for men transitioning through male menopause, sometimes called andropause.

Natural estrogen is available in tablet form by prescription only.

Testosterone

Testosterone is referred to as the female and male sex hormone. Although women produce about one-tenth the level as men, it is responsible for a healthy libido in both sexes. Testosterone also contributes to maintaining the integrity of the skin, muscle, and bones. The amount of testosterone released by the testes in men and the ovaries in women is regulated by the pituitary gland. Levels in men begin to decline anywhere between the ages of thirty and fifty, and may cause a loss of sexual desire, mood swings, irritability, and an increase in the risk of heart disease. This hormonal decline in men is similar to what happens with women during menopause when their ovaries start to deteriorate and the aging cycle begins.

Natural testosterone is available for use, as is synthetic testosterone, although the latter appears to result in more problems than natural hormones. Men over age fifty can have tremendous improvement with testosterone therapy. Numerous studies have shown that testosterone therapy increases strength and muscle mass significantly, improves physical balance, raises red blood cell count, lowers cholesterol, and reduces angina. The amount of testosterone in the body is associated with several health risks. Lower levels are correlated with increased incidents of heart attack and angina. In contrast, higher levels have been found to lower the risk of heart attack, and the more testosterone in the body, the greater the levels of protective HDL cholesterol.

There is some speculation that testosterone may increase the risk of prostate enlargement, or benign prostatic hyperplasia (BPH). Although not well understood, it appears that this condition occurs with age and requires the presence of dihydrotestosterone (DHT), a hormone derived from testosterone. Taking the herb saw palmetto or zinc with testosterone therapy will diminish the potential risk, if any, of prostate enlargement.

Testosterone use must be prescribed and supervised by a physician. Testosterone is administered by injection, tablet or gel.

Human Growth Hormone

Human growth hormone (HGH) is secreted by the pituitary gland in the brain. HGH was first used to successfully treat children who, deficient in this hormone, failed to grow. Since then HGH has been found to be one of the key repair hormones in the body. The body needs sufficient stores of HGH in order to regenerate tissue, make new cells, strengthen bones, replace nails, hair, and skin, and maintain healthy brain function. Production of HGH declines with age.

Studies using HGH replacement therapy show it lowers blood pressure significantly. Arteries and veins in people using HGH appear more capable of removing fluid and of enhancing circulation into the brain and throughout the body; they also have a flexibility associated with younger blood vessels. HGH has also been shown to have positive results with AIDS patients who suffer from severe loss of weight and muscle and, in general, with countering increased body fat and decreased bone mass that occurs with age.

HGH is administered by injection and must be prescribed and supervised by a physician. Although growth hormone therapy is expensive, many of our patients receive one shot per month to significantly lower their blood pressure and improve overall well-being.

Melatonin

Melatonin is both a hormone and an amino acid. It is derived from the amino acid tryptophan by the action of two enzymes in the pineal gland, a light-sensitive gland in the brain that is sometimes referred to as our "third eye." Melatonin is secreted cyclically, rising and falling in a twenty-four-hour biological rhythm influenced by the amount of daylight and darkness. Production begins in the evening, sometime between dusk and 8:00 P.M., and peaks at about midnight. Another peak occurs at around 4:00 A.M. and wanes two hours later. Because light suppresses melatonin production, secretion of this hormone goes up in winter, which, in some people, can lead to depression. The body's pattern of melatonin production is similar to that of DHEA and HGH; it is abundant in early years and steadily declines as we age.

Melatonin has several important functions. It plays a major role in the production of estrogen and testosterone, in the regulation of the body's circadian rhythm (the body's twenty-four-hour internal clock), which controls sleep-wake cycles, and as a powerful antioxidant, which prevents harmful oxidation reactions that can lead to heart disease. Melatonin is also thought to lower blood pressure indirectly by its ability to reduce stress and improve sleep. It may also decrease cancer risk and tumor development, by slowing its rate of growth.

Melatonin is relatively benign in nature and low in toxicity. Nevertheless, melatonin supplements in dosages that produce results are very difficult to obtain without a prescription. In some cases, as much as 80 milligrams (mg) to 250 mg are needed to help individuals sleep and to regulate the hormonal cycle. *Note:* Melatonin is best taken around 8:00 P.M. to boost the body's natural production schedule; if taken too late in the evening, you may wake up in the morning feeling as if it is 4:00 A.M., in which case, adjust your timing slightly.

CHAPTER 7

Putting the Program into Practice

The dietary recommendations and supplement protocols in this book work exceptionally well for the vast majority of the people with high blood pressure and elevated cholesterol, but some trial and error will be needed to tailor the program to your specific biochemical needs.

It is very important for both you and your physician to realize that every person is genetically and biochemically unique. Dietary or nutritional regimens have different effects on different people. The influence of diet on blood fat levels, for example, is not predictable for each individual due to different genetic traits. Dietary sodium restriction is generally recommended for those with high blood pressure and, in most cases but not always, reduces blood pressure. Likewise, the dietary cholesterol found in eggs usually does not significantly raise blood cholesterol in most people if the individual is on a proper dietary regimen. Nevertheless, not all people can consume large quantities of eggs without an increase in blood cholesterol.

Whether your cholesterol and blood pressure are high, borderline, or mild, it's a good idea to have a chemical screening before beginning the program. This metabolic profile, or work-up, will allow you and your physician to customize the dietary and supplement recommendations made in this book and, if temporarily needed, your medications.

The following diagnostic tests should be part of a comprehensive screen. All these tests can be done at your healthcare provider's office:

- amino acids profile

- basic metabolic profile

- complete blood count

- DHEA test (if between the ages of fifty and seventy)

- fatty acids levels

- glucose and insulin levels

- hair analysis (to detect mineral deficiencies and the presence of heavy metals)

- IgE, allergy screen

- lipid levels (triglycerides and cholesterol)

- other blood markers (C-reactive protein, fibrinogen, homocysteine, and more)

- red-blood cell trace elements levels (cadmium, chromium, lead, selenium, and zinc)

- stress test (if prescribed by your doctor)

- thyroid test

- vitamin levels

Once you and your physician have the test results in hand, you are ready to get started. Here's a plan for how to go about your day on the No-More Hypertension and Heart Disease Program:

- Between 7 and 10 A.M.: Have your chosen Rainbow Diet breakfast. Take designated A.M. supplements and medications (if any) with water, Anti-Hypertension Shake (for recipe see pages 163–164), or fresh-squeezed juice. If you'll be out all day, prepare some healthy snacks so you don't find yourself next to the vending machine. Work out for thirty to forty-five minutes.

- Between 8:30 and 11:30 A.M.: Break for designated-hypertension relief consisting of mid-morning exercises such as meditation, prayer, biofeedback, or CES for ten to thirty minutes, or at the level you and your doctor have decided on. Eat one to two snacks between breakfast and lunch.

- Between 12 and 3 P.M.: Choose an approved Rainbow Diet lunch. Take your designated midday supplements and drugs, if needed.

- Between 3:30 and 5:30 P.M.: Break for mid-afternoon stress-relief. Engage in some form of relaxation—meditation, prayer, biofeedback, CES—for ten to thirty minutes. Eat one to two snacks between lunch and dinner.

- Between 6 and 8 P.M.: Enjoy your Rainbow Diet dinner of choice. Take designated P.M. supplements.

- Between 8 and 10 P.M.: Take pre-sleep supplements (if any), or use the CES device for relaxation.

- Wake up the next morning refreshed, filled with energy and in a positive mood.

Keep this daily planner in mind as you incorporate the following Five-Step Plan for eliminating drugs and substituting nutritional supplements. The plan is designed for the typical hypertensive, that is, someone with high blood pressure and elevated cholesterol, who is overweight and presently takes drugs to control these conditions. Once your weight is normalized, and your blood pressure and cholesterol reduced, you can switch to the Five-Step Maintenance Plan.

FIVE-STEP PLAN FOR REPLACING DRUGS WITH NUTRITIONAL SUPPLEMENTS

STEP 1. Follow the Rainbow Diet for weight loss of two to four pounds the first week and two pounds a week thereafter.

STEP 2. Take the following supplements daily:

- 7 tablets Dr. Braverman's Heart Formula (4 with breakfast, 3 with dinner) or the content equivalent in another brand. This formula combines in one supplement many of the key vitamins, minerals, amino acids, and antioxidants found to be the most useful for treating high blood pressure and heart disease. Each tablet contains:

Beta-carotene: 1,222 IU	Potassium: 6.7 mg
Chromium: 26.7 mcg	Selenium: 20 mcg
Garlic powder (odorless): 200 mg	Taurine: 200 mg
Magnesium: 50 mg	Vitamin B_6: 50 mg
Molybdenum: 40 mcg	Vitamin C: 40 mg
Niacinamide: 50 mg	Zinc: 4 mg

- 7, 500-mg capsules of high-potency fish oil (4 with breakfast, 3 with dinner), or 3 tablespoons of a high-potency, emulsified, liquid fish oil. Fish oil is available in several flavors. Vegetarian option: an equivalent dose of flaxseed oil.

- 7, 500-mg capsules of GLA from evening primrose oil, borage oil, or black currant oil (4 with breakfast, 3 with dinner).

- 1 tablet, A.M. and P.M., of Dr. Braverman's Magnesium Formula (Formula #4 in Appendix B, or the content equivalent in another brand). Adjust dose to bowel function: decrease if bowels are too loose; increase by 1–2 tablets if constipated.

- 1–3, 10-mg tablets of potassium (with meals), A.M. only.

- 2 tablets Dr. Braverman's Multivitamin and Mineral Formula (Formula #9 in Appendix B, or the content equivalent in another brand). Women should take additional calcium to prevent osteoporosis, especially if they are thin, fair-skinned, or are pre-or postmenopausal.

STEP 3. Taper off medications. Under your doctor's supervision, gradually reduce the dosage of all antihypertensive and/or cholesterol drugs you're taking. Follow the directions below until you are no longer on medication. Usually one to two drugs can be stopped in thirty days. Occasionally, increases in blood pressure may occur in the early stages of drug reversal. See your physician every seven to fourteen days for an evaluation. Phone immediately if any side effects occur.

- If taking a diuretic, stop immediately, unless you are using Lasix (furosemide) or another super-strong diuretic, in which case, cut dose by half and taper off gradually every one to two weeks.

- If not using a diuretic, cut your beta-blocker or alpha-blocker medication by half every one to two weeks.

- If taking an angiotensin drug, reduce dose by one-half or one-third every one to two weeks.

- If taking a calcium channel blocker, reduce dose by one-half or one-third every one to two weeks.

- If taking a central-acting agent, reduce, and substitute for a less dangerous drug such as an ACE inhibitor.

- If taking any type of cholesterol-lowering drug, take medication every other day for two to four weeks, then discontinue.

STEP 4. If your high numbers for cholesterol and blood pressure don't go into low gear—which can sometimes happen if you're taking two to five drugs a day—increase and/or add the following nutrients:

- Increase fish oil by 2 grams daily.

- Increase GLA from primrose oil, borage oil, or black currant oil by 1 gram daily.

- Increase dose of Dr. Braverman's Heart Formula (Formula #1 in Appendix B) by three tablets for a total of 10 tablets daily (5 with breakfast, 5 with dinner).

- Add up to 2,000 mg of niacin in divided doses. High doses of the zero-flush niacin inositol hexonicotinate can usually be taken without side effects, but sometimes a partial flush will occur. Other effective alternatives are 10 mg of policosanol daily or 1,200 mg of red rice yeast twice daily (with breakfast and dinner).

- Add 1,500 of calcium supplement daily in divided doses for women with osteoporosis.

- Add 10 mg of CoQ_{10} daily, especially if you have a history of heart trouble.

- Add 1–3 grams of arginine, especially if your cholesterol is high.

- Add 1–3 grams of tryptophan, especially if you are nervous.

STEP 5. Engage in only light to mild exercise during this phase of drug withdrawal. Use biofeedback and brain-stress controller CES, especially if your high blood pressure is resistant to treatment. Also, consider chelation therapy. Stubborn high blood pressure and cholesterol numbers should decrease using this regimen.

5-STEP MAINTENANCE PROGRAM

Once your weight is normalized and your blood pressure and cholesterol are at healthy levels, shift to the following maintenance program:

STEP 1. Continue to eat according to the Rainbow Diet. Only now you may add an occasional treat, such as a slice of cheese cake.

STEP 2. Continue to exercise. Only now you may switch from mild exercise to a more rigorous and demanding exercise routine. Aim to exercise thirty to forty-five minutes five to six days of the week.

STEP 3. Continue with meditation (or prayer), and/or a stress reduction technique of your choice, twice daily for fifteen to thirty minutes.

STEP 4. Visit with your doctor once every thirty days, or as needed.

STEP 5. Decrease your intake of daily supplements as follows:

- 4 tablets of Dr. Braverman's Heart Formula (or the content equivalent in another brand).
- 4, 500-mg capsules of high-potency fish oil (2 in A.M., 2 in P.M.), or 2 tablespoons of a high-potency, emulsified, liquid fish oil.
- 4, 500-mg capsules of GLA from evening primrose oil, borage oil, or black currant oil (2 in A.M., 2 in P.M.).
- 1 tablet Dr. Braverman's Magnesium Formula (or the content equivalent in another brand).
- 1–3 tablets Dr. Braverman's Calcium Formula (or the content equivalent in another brand).
- 1, 10-mg tablet potassium.
- 1 tablet Dr. Braverman's Multivitamin and Mineral Formula (or the content equivalent in another brand).

WHAT YOU CAN EXPECT

How quickly you are able to normalize your blood pressure and/or cholesterol and are able to obtain your weight loss goal is highly individual. Everyone is different and the drugs you may presently be on, the severity of your elevated blood pressure and cholesterol, your age, and unique metabolism are all factors to take into consideration. Given these variations, in general, here are the changes you can expect to experience on the No-More Hypertension and Heart Disease Program in the upcoming year:

Results in 30 to 90 Days

- Blood pressure brought into acceptable range from 120/80 to 135/85.
- Triglycerides normalized to 200 or less with a decrease of up to 40 to 50 percent.
- Total cholesterol normalized to 200 or less, or a decrease in total cholesterol from 5 to 40 percent; with an increase in HDL to 50 or above, or between 50 and 300 percent.
- One to two diuretics discontinued (except in cases of severe congestive heart failure). Reduction or discontinuance of all beta- and alpha-block-

ers, central-acting agents, calcium channel blockers, ACE inhibitors, and others.

- Liberalization of the Rainbow Diet in many cases.

Results in 90 to 180 Days

- Off most drugs, unless you are taking four to six antihypertensive drugs.
- Total cholesterol as low as 80 to 110, usually about 150 to 180.
- Blood pressure brought in normal range.
- Maintenance of healthy blood pressure.

How to Make Supplements Easier to Swallow

Here are a few important tips for managing and simplifying your supplement regimen:

- Take all designated vitamins at one time—unless indicated otherwise—shortly before, during, or after a meal when they're digested with the greatest efficiency.

- Take fish oil capsules before meals, to eliminate possible belching.

- Take no-flush—or better yet—zero-flush niacin pills before, not after, meals to reduce the potential for skin flushing. In cases of severe flushing reactions, a baby aspirin prevents flushing if taken before the niacin. If discomfort persists, stop taking the niacin and/or consult your physician. Nausea is also an occasional side effect.

- If you have trouble swallowing vitamins, grind them to a powder in a blender or coffee mill and combine with apple sauce or any liquid.

- Need a gadget to remind you it's pill time? Ask your pharmacist about the "Med-Tymer," an electronic pill-container cap that sounds an alarm and flashes a light at vitamin time. Fits most vitamin bottles.

- Find a fishing tackle box or compartmentalized, plastic lure box and stock the compartments with a monthly supply of vitamins. This will reduce your vitamin-taking time to five minutes daily. To keep moisture out and supplements fresh include a dessicant—one of those small pouches commonly found in supplement bottles—in the box.

Results in 6 Months

- Liberalization of the Rainbow Diet for all persons with continued restrictions on carbohydrate intake for those who remain overweight.

Results in 1 Year

- Reduction in the nutrients needed to keep blood pressure down.

- Continued reduction in drugs, if your hypertension was severe.

- Weight loss goals achieved for nearly everyone. For the rest: be persistent, stick with the carbohydrate restriction and an exercise routine.

- Drug-free, robust life maintained with a small group of key nutritional supplements and a wholesome, easy, colorful diet of whole foods.

Virtually no case of high blood pressure, elevated cholesterol, and obesity cannot be helped—and usually solved—through proper nutrition, diet, and lifestyle changes. But don't just take our word for it. In the upcoming chapters, we'll show you ways to measure your progress and proof that the program works.

CHAPTER 8

Tests for Tracking Your Cardiovascular Fitness

C ertain diagnostic tests can be very valuable for monitoring your progress on the No-More Hypertension and Heart Disease Program. Some tests you can do yourself if you have the right device; others use sophisticated equipment and require trained technicians. Although one or more of the following tests may have been used to first diagnose your high blood pressure or type of heart disease, it's a good idea to retake these tests from time to time. Not only will they help you stay on track so you don't backslide and suddenly find your blood pressure and cholesterol creeping back up, they'll also provide you peace of mind with the assurance your cardiovascular system remains in good working order.

BLOOD PRESSURE MONITORING

Your blood pressure is taken with a device called a sphygmomanometer. To measure blood pressure, the cuff is wrapped around the arm and tightened by means of a pump that inflates the cuff and cuts off most of the circulation in the arm. A valve is then released, allowing air to seep out and the cuff to loosen. A stethoscope is placed over the artery located in the crook of the elbow. The pressure on the meter is read when enough air pressure has been released so the pulsing of blood can be heard through the stethoscope (this is systolic, the top number in a blood pressure reading). The bottom number is read when one stops hearing the pulse (this is diastolic, the lower number).

The currently accepted guide to blood pressure readings was presented in Chapter 1 on page 4. To recap those guidelines here: for middle-age adults, blood pressure below 120/80 is in the normal range; 120/80 to 139/89 is considered "borderline," or mildly elevated; 140/90 to 159/99 is considered stage 1 hypertension; and blood pressure equal or greater than 160/100 is stage 2 hypertension.

Keep in mind that blood pressure has a lot of ups and downs. Only when your pressure is frequently and consistently elevated does it become true hypertension. Three separate readings must be taken in a doctor's office before an accurate diagnosis of high blood pressure can be made.

Mechanical and electronic blood pressure kits are also available for at-home use. Mechanical gauges are similar in structure and operation to those used by physicians; the electronic blood pressure device is a digital sphygmomanometer. Kits typically range from $30 to $100 and can be purchased at most medical pharmacies and from medical mail-order suppliers. The best time to determine your blood pressure is before you get up in the morning. Take your pulse for one full minute.

If you do not have a history of hypertension or heart disease, you can monitor your blood pressure as infrequently as every six months to one year. However, if you have a history of high blood pressure or other heart-related condition, you should have your blood pressure checked at each doctor's visit, or once a week if uncontrolled.

TWENTY-FOUR-HOUR BLOOD PRESSURE MONITOR

The twenty-four-hour blood pressure monitor is an exciting new breakthrough in the management of high blood pressure. The monitor measures a person's nighttime and daytime blood pressures, and as such, is able to capture the fluctuations in blood pressure, which occur throughout a twenty-four-hour period and under different stress conditions. A pressure cuff worn on the arm inflates and deflates automatically about three to four times an hour. Each time it records a blood pressure reading that the practitioner will use later to calculate an average. Because it is able to provide a more realistic and accurate blood pressure profile, it is presently regarded as the ultimate in blood pressure monitoring.

Elevated twenty-four-hour blood pressures are very predictive of the risk for left ventricular hypertrophy (LVH). This means that as blood pressure increases, the heart muscles have to work against more blood pressure, and consequently the heart increases in size. An enlarged heart muscle is not good; just as a person with large biceps is unable to pitch a baseball because of an overly muscular arm, so too do you have to watch out for your heart becoming overly muscular as a result of high pressure. The strain on the heart caused by LVH is one of the main problems associated with sudden death in heart disease. Diagnosis of this condition may require an echocardiogram, in addition to an electrocardiogram. (See information on these two tests later in the chapter.) Fortunately, LVH is a reversible condition in many individuals.

The twenty-four-hour blood pressure monitor is also used to help the doctor monitor the blood-pressure-lowering effects of drug therapy and the effects of a nutritional diet and healthful lifestyle program.

CHOLESTEROL TESTING

Make sure to get an accurate reading of your cholesterol levels. The most accurate cholesterol test is one in which a blood sample is drawn from the vein by a doctor or technician and processed in a hospital or commercial clinical laboratory. The test measures the ratio of your LDL or "bad" cholesterol to HDL or "good" cholesterol. For the most accurate test results, fast for twelve hours. The longer you wait to take the test after eating, the better.

There are also "instant" cholesterol tests, which can be used to check your total cholesterol level at home. Typically, a drop of blood is obtained with a finger prick and placed on a pad containing chemicals that react with your blood and change its color. The color is then compared against a color-coded chart, which indicates your total cholesterol level. These widely available, over-the-counter-cholesterol kits are useful, but they cannot provide as precise a measurement as a lab test.

The currently accepted guide to cholesterol readings was presented in Chapter 1 on page 12. To recap that information here: for middle-age adults, any total cholesterol less than 200 is healthy; 200 to 239 is considered "borderline" and may require treatment if you have other heart disease risk factors; 240 or above makes you a candidate for therapy right away. Cholesterol levels are expressed in milligrams per deciliter of blood, abbreviated as mg/dL (a deciliter is one-tenth of a liter). If your level is high, have another test a week or two later, then base your treatment on the average of the two numbers.

Typically there are three numbers in a cholesterol reading: your total cholesterol (LDL plus HDL) and your LDL and HDL, listed separately. HDL takes cholesterol away from the heart and thereby protects against cancer and heart disease. HDL levels of 60 or greater are good, but the higher your levels of HDL the better. HDL levels of 70 to 80 show extremely low heart disease risk. HDL levels between 15 and 30 indicate trouble, even perhaps a shortened life. The best cholesterol profile is one that has a ratio of low level of LDL cholesterol to a high level of HDL cholesterol. Blood cholesterol readings over 260 quadruple your risk of developing heart disease (compared to levels of 170 or below).

If you have hypertension and/or heart disease, your blood cholesterol levels should be measured twice a year or more by your doctor until they normalize.

USEFUL SUPPLEMENTARY BLOOD TESTS

You may want to include other key markers in a blood screen that can indicate your risk of cardiovascular disease. We mentioned them briefly in Chapter 1 and include them again here:

- C-reactive protein (CRP)
- Fibrinogen
- Homocysteine

PULSE RATE

Your pulse rate tells you how well your heart is functioning. When exercising, aim to keep your heart rate in the low to middle area of the training range—this is about 70 to 75 percent of your aerobic capacity. To determine that range, subtract your age from 220 and multiply the result by .60 and .75. The result is the range for your target number of beats per minute. Check your pulse two to three times throughout your exercise session.

AGE	TARGET ZONE	AGE	TARGET ZONE
20	120–150	50	102–127
25	117–146	55	99–120
30	114–142	60	96–120
35	111–138	65	93–116
40	108–135	70	90–113
45	105–131	75	87–109

Exercise that sustains this target zone level for thirty minutes should be undertaken at least three times and, optimally, up to six times a week. If your pulse rate is over 120 when you stop exercising, it's a sign that your routine was too intense or too long (unless you are young enough that your doctor says it's okay). If your pulse rate is that high, lighten up on the intensity of your exercise. And always do cool-down exercises.

Apart from a rapid pulse brought on by exercise—unnatural lows or highs in blood pressure are associated with a rapid pulse. Hence, another index of how dangerous your high blood pressure is (especially in the diastolic range of 90–95 or systolic 140–160) is your pulse rate. Rapid pulse (greater than 90) can indicate high blood pressure or heart disease that needs further treatment.

Electronic pulse meters are available for $40 to $120 at most sporting goods shops and are easy to use while exercising.

DEXA SCAN

The DEXA Scan (dual energy X-ray absorptionmetry) is a simple, safe, precise, whole-body method of measuring bone density and body composition (fat mass vs. lean mass). Although this technique is most widely used to identify perimenopausal and postmenopausal women with low-bone density, who are most at risk for osteoporosis and fractures, it is becoming more commonplace as a tool for developing therapeutic interventions for the overweight and obese. A DEXA scan measures both total and regional fat mass and, as such, when you are on a weight-loss or improved fitness program, can provide a far more accurate assessment of the actual makeup of the body than simply weighing oneself.

HEART SMARTS: *Did You Know That . . .*

- The thumb has a pulse of its own. That's why you use the index and middle fingers instead of the thumb to take your pulse. In some cases, pulse is a marker of heart health. Rapid pulse (greater than 90) can indicate hypertension or heart disease that needs further treatment.

- The average heart rate is 72.

- Certain colors make you feel better and improve your blood pressure readings. It's not our vision of the color that affects us, but the waves of electromagnetic energy that make up the colors. In one study, changing the colors in a classroom of handicapped children reduced blood pressure. Blue and green are the most relaxing and calming colors; red and yellow the most stimulating.

- Red earlobes or a red nose can sometimes indicate circulatory problems.

- If the visible, light blue blood vessels on the back of your hand are soft and pulsating, it means your cardiovascular system is in good working order.

Body fat measurements can help a person who wishes to lose weight determine how to diet and exercise in order to achieve their weight loss goals. Body fat is the reserve energy stored within body cells. This energy is measured in calories. For every 3,500 calories consumed above the amount expended, the body creates one pound of fat. Lean body mass, on the other hand, is fat-free weight composed of muscle, vital organs, body fluids, connective, and other nonfat tissue. The greater the amount of muscle, the more efficiently the body metabolizes or "burns" fat.

Dieting without exercise, for example, can result in the loss of 50 percent fat and 50 percent muscle, thus maintaining the same ratio of body fat to lean body mass (loss of muscle while dieting is a serious problem and can affect your heart muscle). Looks can be deceiving. Many individuals who appear to still be overweight while dieting will actually have added muscle and lost fat. On the other hand, individuals who appear to be the correct height and weight may actually have too much fat. The scale cannot provide this type of information. A DEXA scan can help tell whether or not a person actually is "redistributing," that is, adding muscle and losing fat.

The body's fat composition changes throughout life. The average American typically loses muscle and gains fat steadily after age twenty, as the following numbers illustrate:

| | PERCENTAGE OF BODY FAT | | | | PERCENTAGE OF BODY FAT | |
AGE	MALE	FEMALE	AGE	MALE	FEMALE
20	10%	19%	40	21%	30%
25	13%	22%	45	22%	31%
30	16%	24%	50	24%	33%
35	19%	28%	55	25%	34%

As we age we all gain body fat. And, although a person may weigh the same at age sixty five as at age thirty, the body may have deteriorated substantially in terms of muscle mass. This does not have to be so. Body muscle can be built up at any age if proper exercise and diet are followed.

During a DEXA scan the patient lays on a table with an open-air covering. Overhead, an x-ray device passes over the body twice using high-speed, low-dose x-rays to capture information. Depending on the purpose for the scan, this data is then used to analyze the mineral content of the bones or the ratio of fat and lean muscle mass in specific areas throughout the body. Using this information, patient and physician can learn what in the diet and exercise regime may or may not be working. The DEXA scan not only calculates the mass ratios, but also predicts the risk of cardiovascular disease and supplies specific suggestions for exercise and weight reduction.

The following is an example of a patient's body fat map. The far left column indicates the area of focus, the second column gives, by grams, the amount of fat in that area, and the third column lists, by grams, the amount of lean muscle mass or bone mineral content. The far right column provides the percentage of fat in a given spot on the body, derived by measuring the grams of fat compared to the grams of lean muscle mass.

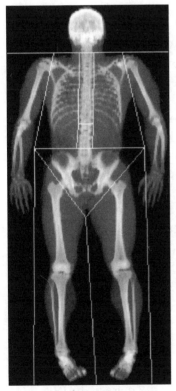

Body Fat Map

DEXA SCAN INFORMATION

Patient name: XX

Sex: M	**Enthnicity:** Caucasian
Current Height: 5'10"	**Current Weight:** 170 lbs
Date of Birth: 12/28/57	**Age:** 47

Region	Fat (grams)	Lean + BMC (grams)	Fat (percent)
L Arm	416.93	4,062.68	9.31
R Arm	405.59	4,576.43	8.14
Trunk	4,377.02	30,651.87	12.50
L Leg	1,263.73	11,456.09	9.94
R Leg	1,390.72	11,841.00	10.51
Subtotal	7,853.99	62,588.07	11.15
Head	902.43	4,055.35	18.20
TOTAL	8,756.42	66,643.42	11.61

The ideal amount of body fat for an adult man is about 8–18 percent and 18–25 percent for an adult woman. Women's bodies naturally carry more fat than men's to ensure that there will always be sufficient internal resources for pregnancy and nursing. The box to the left lists the ranges of percents used to indicate your level of body fat. Aim to maintain your body fat in the low- to average-fat range.

FAT STATUS	Percent Body Fat	
	WOMEN	MEN
Very low fat	9–17	6–10
Low fat	18–21	11–15
Average	22–25	16–18
Above average	26–29	19–20
High fat	30–35	21–25
Very high fat	>35	>25

DEXA scans can be repeated at six-month intervals until you reach your weight/exercise goal. When repeated biannually, it provides you with a "moving picture" of your progress. This method is gaining wide acceptance by sports trainers, exercise physiologists, and nutritionally oriented physicians.

DOPPLER TEST

The Doppler Test is used to determine how well the blood is circulating throughout your cardiovascular system. It uses an advanced computerized instrument to accurately measure the pressure, or volume of blood, flowing throughout the entire circulatory system, including the hands, feet, legs, arms, and neck. From these readings, sites of blood vessel blockages can be identified. Individuals particularly at risk are hypertensives, diabetics, smokers, victims of stroke and transient ischemic attacks (TIAs, or small strokes), the elderly, the overweight, and women who are pregnant.

Depending on which arteries or veins are affected, pain in the legs, cramps, non-healing ulcers, leg swelling, varicosities, numbness, impotence, and a pale skin color are a few of the many early signs of blockages and restricted blood flow. However, symptoms of blockages and restricted blood flow manifest themselves differently, depending on where they occur in the body. If you have one or more of the following symptoms or conditions, having a Doppler Test could provide you with additional valuable information (symptoms that are followed by an asterisk are considered the most common indicators):

Circulation in the Arteries

Bone fractures of the lower extremities

Cigarette smoking

Coldness in an extremity

Diabetes

Diminishing/absent distal or pedal

pulses* (weak pulse in the legs and/or feet)

Distal extremity hair loss* (hair loss typically on the lower legs)

Weakness or fatigue in an extremity*

Frostbite (cold injury)

Heart disease

High blood pressure

Intermittent claudication (cramplike pain in the legs brought on by walking)

Numbness in an extremity

Raynaud's phenomenon (constriction and spasm of the blood vessels in the extremities, resulting in intermittent attacks of pallor of the hands or fingers brought on by emotional stress or frostbite)

Rest pain (pain in the legs without exertion), night cramps*

Skin color changes or ulceration*

Skin or nail infections

Subclavian steal syndrome (a decrease in blood supply to the posterior of the brain due to an occlusion, or obstruction, in the subclavian artery, a major artery of the upper extremities that passes beneath the clavicle bone, which "steals" blood from the vertebral artery leading to the brain)

Thoracic outlet syndrome (pallor of the fingers on elevation of the extremity, sensitivity to cold, or arm claudication due to decreased circulation caused by compression of the subclavian artery between the two neck muscles and clavicle bone or between the upper rib and clavicle bone)

Circulation in the Cerebral/Carotid Arteries

Amaurosis fugax (a loss of vision due to a circulatory problem)

Aphasia (loss of ability to coordinate muscular movement due to a loss of comprehension or productivity using spoken and/or written language)

Ataxia (deterioration of the cerebellum, the part of the brain controlling coordination)

Carotid bruit* (an abnormal sound heard in the carotid artery)

Cluster-type headaches*

Dizziness

Drop attacks (sudden muscular weakness)

Dysarthria (an inability to articulate when speaking caused by a lesion in the brain stem, cerebellum and/or other parts of the brain)

Fluctuating confusion

Increased vessel wall rigidity found during palpitation*

Lapse or loss of memory

Loss of balance

Loss of vision

Motor deterioration

RIND (a reversible ischemic neurologic deficit, such as visual disturbance, muscle weakness, or numbness in an extremity or aphasia due to a temporary occlusion of some vessel in the brain, when complete recovery requires more than twenty-four hours)

Stroke

Syncope (a temporary loss of consciousness)

Unilateral paresthesias (abnormal sensation on one side of the body)

Vertigo*

Visual disturbances

Circulation in the Veins

Oral contraceptive use

Cellulitis

Weakness or fatigue of the extremities*

Presence of pitting edema* (accumulation of fluid in the leg that yields when pressure is applied)

Pulmonary embolism (a blood clot in the lung arteries)

Skin color changes* (darkening of the skin)

Ulcers

Varicose veins* with symptoms such as heaviness in the leg, aching, bleeding, or localized discomfort

Venous thrombosis* (a blood clot in a vein) and postphlebitic syndrome* (edema, ulceration, and pigmentation in the ankle)*

No special preparation is needed before taking the Doppler test. The examination is safe and painless. You may be asked to change into a loose-fitting gown in order to make it easier to perform the required measurements. During it, the patient is asked to remain quiet and refrain from talking. Blood pressure cuffs are placed on the area to be tested and small probes are taped to the fingers and toes. The blood pressure cuff is then inflated and rotated and the visual information about the arteries and veins is transferred via infrared light waves and ultrasound (high-frequency sound waves used to record light reflections), which appear on a strip chart or televisionlike screen. From these wave formations it is possible to determine if blockages or clots are present, and where. There are absolutely no needles used and the procedure is completely painless. The entire test may take about an hour since such extensive and thorough readings are needed. In the high-quality machines, a color picture will be available for your review.

For the most accurate results, tobacco, caffeine, and other vascular constrictors should not be used for twenty-four hours prior to testing. Cold hands or feet can also produce falsely abnormal readings, as can tension and movement.

Many diseases require this type of extensive vascular study. Some of the conditions caused by circulation troubles include heart disease, peripheral vascular disease, high blood pressure, Raynaud's syndrome, impotence, intermittent claudication, ischemic ulcers, strokes, kidney failure, leg gangrene, phlebitis, varicose veins, leg edema (or swelling), and cold hands or feet. Some of these conditions are more dangerous than others; some symptoms are visible and some are not. For example, in the atherosclerotic process, the body is gradually starved of oxygen due to insufficient circulation. Sometimes symptoms such as chest pain or leg cramps (especially in the cold or after walking) can be symptoms of this process. Most of the time, however, there is no way to detect the process until it is so advanced that a serious medical problem results. The Doppler Test is one of the few ways to detect early signs of blood vessel disease before it causes any damage.

The Doppler Test can be done once or twice a year or more often if severe heart disease or peripheral vascular disease is present.

ELECTROCARDIOGRAM AND ECHOCARDIOGRAM

An electrocardiogram (EKG) is a diagnostic test that provides a printout of the electrical activity of the heart. It measures whether or not your heart is working efficiently or if there is an electrical conduction delay resulting in uneven heart muscle contraction. It can tell whether the different chambers of your heart are working in rhythm with each other, or are "out of sync." All sorts of irregular beats and their causes can be detected with an EKG. An EKG is also valuable for detecting whether you have had a "silent" (symptomless) heart attack in the past and can show if there are signs of an impending one. Finally, an enlarged or hypertrophied heart muscle may show up as an abnormal tracing. The test is noninvasive and involves the placement of electrodes on the chest and extremities, which then conduct the electrical information back through the electrocardiograph and onto paper.

A normal EKG can be a great reassurance that your heart is functioning well and working harmoniously with your body to contribute to your good health. This is especially true when the EKG is accompanied by an echocardiogram.

An echocardiogram is a test that uses ultrasound to compile a picture of the heart valves and their functionality. It shows the heart size and its pumping efficiency, and can reveal any structural or functional abnormalities. The echocardiogram, along with a positron emission tomography test (see following), is an effective way to accurately assess subtle heart disease not detected by an EKG.

Every adult over the age of thirty should have an EKG once a year and adults at high risk, twice a year.

HOLTER MONITOR

The Holter monitor is a small devise worn on the body that measures the rhythms of the heartbeat over a twenty-four-hour period. A continuous recording of the heart's rhythms enables a physician to distinguish among the many different types of arrhythmias with their varying degrees of severity. It can detect subtle arrhythmias that would otherwise go unnoticed and life-threatening arrhythmias, thus also helping a physician decide which medication, or even which nutritional approach, might help. It frequently detects sick sinus syndrome, a condition in which the heart beats dangerously slow. People with this condition need a pacemaker. Any person with a potential cardiac arrhythmia history should utilize a Holter monitor.

POSITRON EMISSION TOMOGRAPHY

Positron emission tomography (PET) is a test used to assess blood flow through the arteries to the heart without a catheter or dye. This procedure involves injecting positive electrons that have been immersed in a glucose solution into the arteries. Over a two-hour period a series of 130 x-rays are taken. The PET scan detects approximately 50 percent of low-level blockages in the blood vessels. Although not ideal due to radiation exposure from the x-rays (even though minimal), it is far better than waiting for blockages in the circulation to reach 75 to 90 percent, a level detected by more conventional, costly, and time-consuming techniques such as coronary angiography and the stress test.

Because of the increased risk of heart disease after age fifty, consider having a PET scan once every three to five years.

CHAPTER 9

Proof of the Program: Twenty-Five Case Histories

The proof of any high blood pressure and heart disease program is the number of cardiovascular disease sufferers who are returned to a normal daily life with their condition under control or reversed. A top-notch program does even more: It prevents the disorder from recurring. The No-More Hypertension and Heart Disease Program will do both for you if you give it your all. Even if you follow the program halfheartedly, you'll be rewarded.

The following case histories are compiled from actual patient charts. These twenty-five examples are pooled from thousands of records for people whom we have treated and cured of heart disease. They read like a physician's notes with short, to-the-point facts. The numbers speak for themselves. They are proof our program works.

When a patient first comes to our clinic for treatment, he or she receives a complete diagnostic, risk-factor assessment, and a comprehensive exam of the body's cardiovascular system from which we devise a course of action. The first set of case histories profiles people who obtained results using the diet and supplement alone. The second set includes case histories for those whose heart disease was initially resistant to treatment but was ultimately successful with the addition of chelation therapy and stress-reduction techniques.

CASE HISTORIES TREATED WITH DIET AND SUPPLEMENTS

The following case histories illustrate the ability of diet and supplements to treat a broad range of patients regardless of the severity of their high blood pressure and heart disease, their weight and lifestyle habits, and the number of medications they were taking.

Case 1: Reduction of Three Out of Four Prescriptions

G.F. is a fifty-year-old male on multiple medications, 6'0", weighing 265 pounds with a twenty-five-year history of smoking two packs of cigarettes a day. He quit smoking three years ago. His blood pressure was 140/100 with a pulse of 74. He had been taking 250 mg of Aldomet (methyldopa) for hypertension, 40 MEq of Klotrix (a prescription potassium supplement), and 37.5 mg of Dyazide (hydrochlorothiazide/triamterene), a potassium-sparing thiazide diuretic, for ten years. He also used Nitro-Dur (a nitroglycerin patch) nightly to help control his blood pressure.

G.F. was put on the Rainbow Diet and started on a daily regimen of six multivitamins; vitamin B_6 (500 milligrams [mg]); of magnesium orotate (3 grams [g]); of garlic (1,440 mg); of taurine (3 g); of primrose oil (3 g); of Max-EPA (eicosapentaenoic acid, 6 g); of magnesium oxide (1.5 g); and Klotrix (40 MEq). Aldomet was reduced to one tablet and Dyazide was reduced by half.

After one month, his blood pressure had slightly increased to 144/104 (not uncommon with early reversal drugs), but his weight had dropped to 248 pounds. By the next visit, his blood pressure was 120/88, pulse 70, and his weight was 249 pounds. Aldomet was tapered off and Dyazide was stopped. Several weeks later, his blood pressure had again increased; this time to 140/90, his pulse was 78, and his weight was 235 pounds. But he still used Nitro-Dur and Klotrix.

One month later, G.F's blood pressure was 140/94 with a pulse of 70 and his weight was 226. At this point the taurine was reduced to 3 g and garlic to 960 mg. He was no longer on any medication except for the Nitro-Dur and Klotrix. Klotrix was reduced to one tablet, and fish oil was switched to Mega-EPA, a more potent brand of EPA. Two zinc pills (25 mg); magnesium oxide was substituted for magnesium orotate (1,000 mg); and niacin (1 g) were added to the supplement plan. Two tablespoons of safflower oil daily were also prescribed.

At his next check-up, his blood pressure was 150/90, pulse 78, and weight 216. Vitamin C (2 g) was added to his daily supplements.

Over the next four weeks his blood pressure dropped to 130/70, pulse 80, and he lost two more pounds. The Nitro-Dur was stopped. Supplementation was reduced to four multivitamins; 60 mg garlic; 2 g taurine; 2 g primrose oil; 6 g Mega-EPA; and his antihypertensive formula was stopped. One tablet of chromium (200 mcg) was added.

Over a period of several months, G.F. was completely removed from drugs. His blood pressure remains stable at 130/70 with a pulse of 78. His cholesterol was 290 and triglycerides were 280, but three months later dropped to 223 and 122, respectively. He occasionally drinks vodka, coffee, and tea. His sex drive increased gradually throughout the treatment and his exercise intensity (walking) gradually increased.

Case 2: Sky-High Hypertension Lowered in Seven Weeks

D.B., a fifty-one-year-old female with a ten-year history of high blood pressure, migraine headaches, and atrophic vaginitis was presented to us for treatment. She weighed 150 pounds at 5'3", and was taking Lopressor (metoprolol, 50 mg) A.M. and P.M. for her blood pressure. She did not smoke or drink alcohol or tea. Her blood pressure was 194/120, with a pulse of 116.

She began taking two multivitamins; vitamin B_6 (500 mg); folic acid (60 mg) for atrophic vaginitis (vaginal dryness due to aging and loss of sex hormones, especially estrogen); magnesium oxide (2 g) for migraine; taurine (3 g); garlic (1,440 mg); Mega-EPA (6 g); and six antihypertensive heart formula pills.

At D.B's next checkup, her blood pressure was 160/100 with a pulse of 92, and she had not had a migraine in the previous three weeks, the longest period of time she had been migraine-free in years. Her regimen was adjusted to 3 g of magnesium oxide; 2 g taurine; 600 mg calcium carbonate; 3 g primrose oil; 100 mg niacin; 200 mcg chromium; 200 mcg selenium; and 50 mg Lopressor with instructions to taper off the Lopressor if there was improvement in two weeks.

She returned one month later drug-free, and her blood pressure was 130/80 with a pulse of 86. The rapid recovery of this patient was due to following a modified version of the Rainbow Diet that included fish two times daily, lean meat two to three times a week, 3 tablespoons of safflower oil daily, and the frequent use of ginger, garlic and onions.

Case 3: Return of Healthy Blood Pressure after Thirty Years

C.H., a fifty-seven-year-old male, 5'6", weighing 166 pounds, came to us for treatment with a thirty-year history of high blood pressure. At this point, his blood pressure was 160/100 with a pulse of 68, his triglycerides were 256, his cholesterol 190, and he had a HDL fraction of 26 (indicating high coronary risk). He was taking Corgard (nadolol, 20 mg) for high blood pressure, had a moderate sex drive, and did not use caffeine; he also did not exercise.

He started on two GTF chromium (200 mcg, A.M. and P.M.); vitamin C (1 g, A.M. and P.M.); 10 drops of Ziman (a combination of 10 mg of zinc and 2 mg of manganese); selenium (200 mcg, A.M. only); molybdenum (40 mcg); Max-EPA (6 g); taurine (500 mg); magnesium orotate (2 g); and his blood pressure medication was reduced to 10 mg a day.

One month later, a time-release form of niacin was added. His weight had fallen to 154 pounds and his blood pressure was 120/75.

At his next checkup, the Corgard was reduced to 10 mg every other day, and he was advised to stop it in two weeks. One tablespoon of safflower oil A.M. and P.M. was added; 50 mg of zinc A.M. and P.M.; and all other supplements remained the same.

Several weeks later, C.H. complained of feeling light-headed. His blood pressure was 85/70 with a pulse of 90. Medication remained the same (he had forgotten to stop taking the Corgard as instructed), but the safflower oil was stopped. His triglycerides were normal at 153, with cholesterol of 176 and an HDL fraction of 41 with all drugs removed.

When he returned one month later he had a blood pressure of 132/62, pulse of 66, and weighed 149 pounds.

Case 4: Stabilization of a Risky Lipid Profile

N.K., a fifty-three-year-old male, 5'11-½", weighing 209 pounds with a fifteen-year history of high blood pressure, came to us for treatment. He was taking the following blood pressure medications daily: Maxzide (hydrochlorothiazide/triamterene, 25/ 37.5 mg), Lopressor (300 mg), and Minipress (prazosin, 20 mg). He was also taking Zyloprim (allopurinol, 300 mg) for the treatment of gout. He had a moderate sex drive, drank two cups of coffee a day, and had as many as three to seven drinks a week. His blood pressure was initially 130/85, his pulse 66. His triglycerides were 327, HDL 46, and he had a high cholesterol level of 255 with an LDL count of 146.

N.K. was started on one multivitamin a day and prescribed to take the following supplements morning and evening: GTF chromium (200 mcg); time-release niacin (400 mg); a vitamin C, calcium, and magnesium powder (1 to 2 teaspoons); magnesium oxide (500 mg); taurine (500 mg); methionine (500 mg); two Mega-EPA (1 g); and zinc (15 mg). Vitamin B_6 (500 mg) was taken in the morning only. He reduced his dosage of Maxzide to every other day and was instructed to stop it if light-headedness developed. Because he was overweight and had harmful trigylceride levels, he was asked to go on a carbohydrate-deprivation diet and a protein and vegetable diet with no bread or fruit.

By his follow-up visit, N.K.'s blood pressure had dropped to 118/78, his pulse to 60, and his weight to 196 pounds. As per a phone consultation, during this period he reduced his A.M. and P.M. doses of Lopressor to 100 mg and of Minipress to 5 mg. Maxzide was stopped altogether based on blood pressure readings done at home. His intake of vitamin C and magnesium oxide was reduced due to diarrhea and, except for the addition of 200 mcg of selenium, the other supplements remained virtually the same but with increases in the morning and nightly doses for GTF chromium (200 mcg); Mega-EPA (3 g); primrose oil (1 g); and taurine (1 g); zinc (15 mg, A.M.) and (30 mg, P.M.); and two multivitamins. Niacin was increased to three times a day, or 1,200 mg.

One month later, N.K. returned with a blood pressure of 120/80, weight 188, triglycerides now normal at 200, cholesterol reduced to 238, LDL reduced to 134, and HDL increased to 51. His intake of Minipress had now gradually been reduced to 2.5 mg a day, and Lopressor to 100 mg every other day. The supplement regimen was adjusted to zinc (15 mg; A.M., 30 mg P.M.), and to two multivitamin tablets in the morning and evenings. For slight depression, one tablet of the trace mineral lithium was prescribed for use at nighttime along with 500 mg of tryptophan, (A.M. and P.M.). Methionine was reduced to 100 mg (A.M. and P.M.), and niacin to twice a day. Magnesium oxide was stopped due to continued problems with diarrhea.

Over the next four weeks, N.K. dropped his blood pressure and weight even further. His weight was now 184, and he had a blood pressure reading of 110/80. His pulse was 75. He was now put on Lopressor (50 mg) every other day.

By N.K.'s next visit, he was drug-free and had blood pressure of 120/80 consistently over multiple readings.

Case 5: A Sixty-Point Drop in Blood Pressure

M.L., a sixty-five-year-old female, 5'6", weight 170, with a long history of high blood pressure, was presented to us. She was being treated with diuretics, had a blood pressure reading of 170/110, pulse of 102, triglycerides 70, and total cholesterol 234 (LDL 138, HDL 65). She was placed on a low-carbohydrate version of the Rainbow Diet and a supplement regimen. This included: GTF chromium (200 mcg, A.M. and P.M.), niacin timed-release (2 g, A.M. and 1 g, P.M.); vitamin B_6 (500 mg, A.M.), vitamin E (400 IU, A.M. and P.M.); vitamin A (24,000 IU, A.M.); selenium (200 mcg, A.M.); Max-EPA (3 g, A.M./ 2 g at noon/ 3 g, P.M.); tyrosine (2 g, A.M.); methionine (1 g, A.M.); and one Ziman (a combination of 10 mg of zinc and 2 mg of manganese).

M.L. returned one month later with blood pressure of 152/90, a pulse of 88, and weight of 164. She was put on primrose oil (1 gram, A.M. and P.M.), vitamin C (2 ½ g, A.M. and P.M.), safflower oil (1 teaspoon, A.M. and P.M.).

By the next visit her blood pressure was 110/85 without medication, her pulse was 78, and her weight,162. Her blood pressure remains well controlled on this regimen.

Case 6: The Blood-Pressure-Lowering Effect of Supplements

A.F., a forty-five-year-old female, 5'5", 105 pounds, was being treated with Dyazide (25/37.5 A.M. and P.M.) for water retention and Lopressor (50 mg) for hypertension. She had a blood pressure reading of 130/80, with triglyceride and cholesterol readings of 115 and 178, respectively. She started with two multivitamins once a day; GTF chromium (200 mcg, A.M.); time-release niacin (400 mg, A.M. and P.M.); vitamin B_6 (500 mg, A.M.); methionine (500 mg, A.M. and P.M.); tryptophan (1 gram, before sleep); taurine (500 mg, A.M.); primrose oil (1.5 g, A.M. and P.M.); Max-EPA (1 g, A.M. and P.M.); and zinc (15 mg, A.M. and P.M.). Dyazide was reduced to one capsule daily; Lopressor was tapered off.

At her next visit, we recommended A.F. take the Dyazide every other day and stay with the same regimen of vitamins.

Several weeks later her blood pressure was 110/80, pulse 80, and weight 109. She was off all blood pressure medications. In this case, A.F. changed very little in her diet, except for the reduction of fried foods, caffeine, and white flour. This illustrates the strong effect of nutrients, in and of themselves.

Case 7: Improvement with Supplements Only

K.W., a fifty-six-year-old female, 5'10", weight 185, with a ten-year history of high blood pressure came to us. She drank one to two cups of coffee a day and was presented to us with a blood pressure of 160/90, pulse 80, triglycerides 154, and cholesterol 233, taking one Dyazide (25/37.5 A.M. and P.M.) daily. She was started on one multivitamin tablet a day; one tablet of GTF chromium (200 mg, A.M. and P.M.); time-release niacin (400 mg); vitamin B_6 (500 mg, A.M.); taurine (500 mg, A.M. and P.M.); MegaEPA (1 g, A.M. and P.M.); magnesium oxide (50 mg, A.M. and P.M.); and primrose oil (1 g, A.M. and P.M.).

At her next visit, K.W. presented with a blood pressure of 140/84, a pulse of 78, after having stopped her diuretic, with a weight of 181 pounds. At this time she had not yet begun the magnesium or niacin. Later she did, which lowered her cholesterol and triglycerides to 199 and 152, respectively, and her blood pressure to 120/80 with a pulse of 72, a level she has maintained since.

Case 8: Success at Eighty

M.V., an eighty-year-old female, 4'11", 115 pounds, on diuretics for twenty years, drinking four cups of coffee daily, had a blood pressure of 200/98, with a pulse of 88. She was started on two multivitamins; vitamin B_6 (500 mg); calcium pantethine (2 g); zinc (30 mg); manganese (5 mg); magnesium oxide (3 g); calcium orotate (1,500 mg); taurine (3 g); 3 tabs of tyrosine and dl-phenylalanine to help curb her coffee addiction.

Her blood pressure at her follow-up visit was 180/90 and her pulse was 78. Supplementation was upped to four multivitamins a day and 30 mg of zinc twice daily. Manganese was stopped. Calcium was reduced to 1 g. Two grams of primrose oil were added, as well as 3 g of vitamin C and 2,000 mg of fish oil (EPA).

One month later, her blood pressure was 174/80, pulse 76, and weight was stable at 113.5 pounds. The taurine was reduced to 2 g. The primrose oil was increased to 3.5 g, vitamin C to 5 g, and fish oil to 3 g. After several weeks on this regimen her blood pressure dropped to 150/90. Her pulse remained at 76, and she gained 2.5 pounds. One tablespoon of safflower oil was added along with 1 g of magnesium. At this point, she was removed from diuretics.

Four weeks later, her blood pressure dropped to 150/80, and she had lost 1.5 of the 2.5 pounds she had gained.

Case 9: High Blood Pressure Down, Energy and Sex Drive Up

J.K. was a sixty-two-year-old man with a ten-year history of high blood pressure. He had a total cholesterol level of 264, his triglycerides were 161, and his HDL and LDL were 59 and 158, respectively. He was taking 100 mg of Normodyne (labetalol) twice a day for his hypertension, Dyazide (25/37.5 mg), and Lopid (gemfibrozil, 600 mg, A.M. and P.M.) for lowering cholesterol. He was taken off all three drugs in two weeks. Because he presented initially with a blood pressure of 140/90, and was 136 pounds at 5'3", he was put on a modified version of the Rainbow Diet that was lower in carbohydrates and higher in protein.

For his treatment he was prescribed eight primrose oil pills (500 mg); 6 Mega-EPA (1 g); 2 teaspoons liquid fish oil; 6 tablets of our Heart Formula (#1); one tablet of our Magnesium Formula (#4), along with 200 mg of a niacin-garlic formula (Niagar). Initially, in the first week, he stopped taking Dyazide and Lopid, and went to half dose of Normodyne, which he discontinued in the second week.

When he returned for a medical appointment two months after his initial visit, his blood pressure was lowered to 120/80. In addition, his weight had fallen from 136 to 131, his total cholesterol levels dropped from 264 to 181, his triglycerides and LDL fell from 161 to 100 and 158 to 97, respectively, and his HDL increased five points from 59 to 64. He was then continued on this program, which also included 3 tablespoons of safflower oil.

He returned the following week with blood pressure of 110/80. Gradually, his supplements were reduced and he was put on the traditional version of the Rainbow Diet and is still doing exceptionally well, and is completely drug-free. His energy level and sex drive have increased enormously.

Case 10: Blood Pressure and Kidney Function Improved

J.B., a fifty-four-year-old, 6'2", 175-pound man with a diagnosis of high blood pressure and renal insufficiency (inadequate or impaired kidney function) came to us for treatment. His total cholesterol was 176 and his HDL was 44. He was placed on six capsules of Mega-EPA (500 mg); eight capsules of primrose oil (500 mg), six capsules of our Heart Formula (#1); one tablet of our Magnesium Formula (#4), two capsules of niacin-garlic formula (Niagar); one tablet of our Antioxidant Formula (#2); and N-acetyl-cysteine (500 mg). He was initially on Lopressor (50 mg) and the diuretic Hydrodiuril (hydrochlorothiazide, 25 mg).

Within two weeks he had tapered off both drugs, and despite this quick cut back, his blood pressure had fallen from 140/90 to 140/85.

Two-and-a-half months later, his cholesterol had fallen to 130 and his blood pressure was 130/82, on average, and he was completely drug-free. Initial elevations in a substance indicative of kidney function called creatinine fell from 1.7 to 1.3, and he is still doing fine a year later, drug-free on basically the same regimen. His energy level and sex drive have increased enormously.

Case 11: Sharp Drop in Lipids and Surge in Well-Being

G.W., a fifty-five-year-old female with a five-year history of high blood pressure was taking Lozol (indapamide, 2.5 mg) for hypertension and fluid retention. Her total cholesterol was 250, her triglycerides 639, she weighed 159 pounds at 5'2", and ran a constant blood pressure of 176/100.

She was put on three tablespoons of fish oil liquid (equivalent to approximately 2,000 mg), which she preferred to large capsules; eight evening primrose oil (500 mg); eight Heart Formula (#1) capsules; 2 g of niacin, as well as two tablespoons of safflower oil and one capsule of Magnesium Formula (#4).

In one month, her triglycerides fell from 639 to 419, her total cholesterol fell from 250 to 225; her HDL level remained stable at about 32; her weight dropped from 159 pounds to 148 pounds; her diuretic was discontinued; and her blood pressure was 140/78. She continues to do extremely well with excellent control of her blood pressure and continued lowering of her cholesterol as she continues to lose weight on a modified version of the Rainbow Diet that is low in carbohydrates and high in protein. When she reaches her ideal weight, she will be switched to the traditional Rainbow Diet plan. Her energy, happiness and sense of well-being have increased dramatically.

Case 12: Advance of Stage 2 Hypertension Halted

H.H., a forty-nine-year-old female with a two-year history of stage 2 hypertension, presented at 5'3", 173 pounds, with blood pressure consistent at 160/100, cholesterol 204. Her triglycerides were good at 75, as was her HDL of 83.

She was placed immediately on a low-carbohydrate, high-protein version of the Rainbow Diet, as well as put on three fish oil capsules (500 mg); six primrose oil capsules (500 mg); two Heart Formula (#1) capsules; two Calcium Formula (#3) capsules, one capsule each of Magnesium Formula (#4), Antioxidant Formula (#2), Brain-Energy Formula (#10), an amino acid combination for energy; as well as 1,500 mg of the niacin-garlic formula (Niagar) and a tryptophan complex for sleep.

Over a period of five weeks, H.H. lost six pounds and her blood pressure fell to 110/79, where it has remained over many months. She continued to lose weight steadily. Three months later, she weighed 147 and had lost twenty-six pounds. Her blood pressure was 110/68. Her blood pressure is still monitored monthly, reading approximately 110/70 consistently. She continues on the modified version of the Rainbow Diet, and once her normal weight is reached, will be switched to the traditional Rainbow Diet plan at which time she will have a reduction in her pills. At this time, H.H.'s energy level, sense of well-being, and mood are at their best in her life.

Case 13: No More Heart Attacks

This case pertains to T.H., a fifty-five-year-old male with a history of heart attack. When he first came to the office, his total cholesterol measured 234, his triglycerides 289, LDL 132, and HDL 30. At 6'2", 172 pounds, he had blood pressure of 140/80 with a pulse of 68. He was resistant to any dietary treatment.

He began the Rainbow Diet and was placed on six fish oil capsules (500 mg); eight capsules primrose oil (500 mg); two multivitamins; four tablets of Heart Formula (#1); and 3 g of niacin. He was also taking Cardizem CD (diltiazem, 240 mg) for high blood pressure, which he began to taper off.

In one month his cholesterol fell from 234 to 180, triglycerides fell from 289 to 179, HDL levels went up to 33, and his blood pressure temporarily increased.

Six weeks later he had an outstanding cholesterol level of 114 with an HDL of 47, and a pulse that had fallen from 68 to 59. With a reduction in supplements, his pulse and blood pressure returned to normal levels permanently. His weight has fallen from 172 to 163, his blood pressure is 108/60, and he remains on the Rainbow Diet. This has resulted in a significant reduction of his vitamin supplement dosages, and he was told to go off the Cardizem. His energy and sense of well-being have greatly improved, and his risk for another heart attack has decreased.

Case 14: Relief from High Blood Pressure, Diabetes, and Depression

This case resulted in the elimination of Normodyne and the angiotensin-converting enzyme inhibitor Vasotec (enalapril), two strong drugs for lowering of blood pressure. D.W., a sixty-four-year-old female with a thirteen-year history of high blood pressure, as well as uncontrolled diabetes and severe depression, was treated daily with 150 mg of Normodyne and 10 mg of Vasotec. Initially, her blood pressure was 170/90.

We started D.W. on a basic supplement regimen of two tablets of Magnesium Formula (#4); four capsules of taurine (500 mg); and six capsules of primrose oil (500 mg). Both drugs were tapered off and her blood pressure temporarily increased one month later to 190/98.

To counteract this rise, we added 6 g of fish oil; an additional 1 g of magnesium; 400 mg of time-release niacin; plus 1 tablespoon of safflower oil daily. We added six Heart Formula (#1) pills.

Seven days later, D.W.'s blood pressure had fallen to 150/82, and three weeks later, it had fallen again to 140/80, where it has remained while on the current supplement program and on a liberalized version of the Rainbow Diet. She is now free of Normodyne and Vasotec. In addition, her depression was relieved significantly and control of diabetes was established.

Case 15: Turning Back a Poor Cardiovascular Profile

In this case, two dangerous drugs were discontinued. It concerns a sixty-eight-year-old man, E.B., 6'1", 177 pounds, with a blood pressure of 120/80 and a pulse of 84. He had a five-year history of high blood pressure and was being treated with the central-acting agent Aldomet (250 mg) twice daily, and one tablet of the diuretic Dyazide (25/37.5 mg).

His initial program consisted of a low carbohydrate/high protein version of the Rainbow Diet, plus vitamin B_6 (500 mg); taurine (2 g); six capsules primrose oil (500 mg); six capsules fish oil (500 mg); time-release niacin (400 mg); and four capsules of methionine (500 mg). The Dyazide was immediately discontinued, and the Aldomet was tapered off and then eliminated one month later. Sixty days later, E.B. had achieved a blood pressure reading of 120/80 without either drug.

Eight months later, his blood pressure was normal; he had an HDL cholesterol reading that increased from 36 to 52, and triglycerides that dropped from 195 to 90. His good cholesterol (HDL) continued to stay essentially the same. Despite discontinuing two dangerous drugs, he had a complete reversal of his poor cardiovascular profile. He was then placed on the traditional Rainbow Diet eating plan.

Case 16: A Slew of Heart Risk Factors Reversed

This case illustrates the healing of depression, high blood pressure of 180/100, reduction of high cholesterol of 220, and other heart risk factors without drugs. A sixty-two-year-old female, K.W., with an eight-year history of high blood pressure, was being treated with 40 mg each of the loop diuretic Lasix (furosemide) and the beta-blocker Visken (pindolol).

She was started on five capsules garlic oil (1,440 mg); six capsules primrose oil (500 mg); six capsules fish oil (500 mg); magnesium (1 g); zinc (30 mg); vitamin B_6 (500 mg); and a multivitamin.

Within thirty days her pressure reading was 130/80 and her total cholesterol was lowered to 170. Immediately, the Lasix was stopped, and within another thirty days her blood pressure had stayed in the good category of 130/80. But when the Visken was tapered off, her blood pressure creeped up to 140/90 (increases in blood pressure can occur in the early stages of drug reversal).

She was then advised to take a total of 8 g of fish oil and 4.5 g of primrose oil. Her blood pressure fell to the safe range of 130/80, where it remains today. Furthermore, her depression has lifted.

Case 17: Unmanageable Hypertension Brought Under Control

J.J. was a fifty-three-year-old male who had wrestled with poorly controlled high blood pressure for fifteen years. When he came to us he was being treated with

Minipress and Lopressor. He was tapered off these three drugs with the simple application of weight loss and a supplement regimen consisting of ten pills a day of the Heart Formula (#1).

Case 18: From High-Risk Hypertention to Low-Risk in Two Months

In this case history, four types of drugs were eliminated and a return of the sex drive was experienced. A forty-nine-year-old man, H.P., with a twenty-year history of high blood pressure and a ten-year history of elevated triglycerides, came to us for help. His daily medications consisted of 250 mg of Lorelco (probucol), an antilipid drug, two times a day; 50 mg of Lopressor twice a day; 100 mg of the vasodilator Apresoline (hydralazine) three times a day; 25/37.5 mg of Dyazide; and 200 mg of Anturane (sulfinpyrazone) twice daily, which was protecting him from gout caused by his diuretic. On medication, H.P.'s blood pressure was 150/95. He was asymptomatic at that time, although his sex drive was greatly diminished.

We immediately stopped his Lorelco because we knew that we could substitute fish oil for the Lorelco-type drugs. We also stopped the Anturane. We put him on 8 capsules of fish oil (500 mg); primrose oil (3 g); magnesium (1 g); carnitine (1 g); vitamin B_6 (500 mg), and some multivitamins.

Despite putting him on the Rainbow Diet, this 5'9.5", 164-pound man had lost only two pounds when he returned eleven days later with a blood pressure of 130/90.

During this visit we added 2 g of taurine; 1 g of garlic; 30 mg of zinc; and 400 mg of time-released niacin to his program. We also included nutrients such as GTF chromium, selenium, and inositol. We reduced the Lopressor to 25 mg twice a day.

In one month, H.P. returned with a blood pressure reading of 120/88. We put him on a low-carbohydrate, high-protein version of the Rainbow Diet, discontinued the Lopressor, and eventually tapered off his dose of the vasodilator Hydralazine, substituting one 5 mg pill of Vasotec, which has fewer side effects.

He returned four weeks later with blood pressure readings between 120–130 over 70–80. His blood pressure was under control. He was off the Lopressor and Apresoline and was just using Vasotec. (Diazide was stopped.) Initially, he had an HDL of 41, triglycerides of 394, and a total cholesterol reading of 205. In two months on this modified version of the diet, his HDL had jumped to 55, his triglycerides had fallen from 394 to 225, and his cholesterol remained essentially the same. Importantly, H.P.'s sex drive was now normal. In addition, there was tremendous improvement in his HDL fraction and a reduction in his triglycerides. Without lipid-lowering drugs, his treatment was a complete success. His current one-pill dosage of Vasotec does not produce any symptoms. Once a high-risk patient for heart disease and stroke, he is now becoming a low-risk patient.

Case 19: Successful Treatment for Heavy Metal Toxicity

E.K., a seventy-two-year-old male, came to us for treatment for carotid blockages and aluminum toxicity. He had chest pain with mid-sternal chest pressure on exertion, radiating to the left arm accompanied by shortness of breath, that was relieved only by rest. His blood workup revealed an HDL level of 34 and aluminum toxicity. His urine showed both lead and aluminum in excess. Evaluation of his positive emission tomography (PET) scan showed partial death of the heart tissue. Echocardiogram showed he had an ejection fraction of 41 percent. He had left ventricular hypertrophy (LVH) with decreased left ventricular systolic function, dilated aortic root, dilated left atrium and no evidence of any weak valves in the heart. Three years earlier, he had been diagnosed with a blood clot in the lungs, high blood pressure, and high levels of cholesterol and triglycerides. He was also in male menopause (andropause) and had decreased levels of testosterone. These medical problems required extremely close medical supervision.

E.K. was started on a daily supplement plan that included: fish oil (2 g); vitamin D (5,000 mg); choline (500 mg, in A.M. and two in P.M.); safflower oil (1 teaspoon); primrose oil (4 g); time-release niacin (400 mg); pantethine (6 mg); vitamin A (8,500 IU); and carnitine (1 g), as well as the following formulas: Heart Formula (#1); Antioxidant Formula (#2); Calcium Formula (#3); Magnesium Formula (#4); and Brain-Energy Formula (#10). He required close monitoring to ensure he followed the Rainbow Diet.

He is presently taking Nitro ointment (1") applied twice daily; Cardizem CD (240 mg) and Ismo (isosorbide, 20 mg,) for angina; Vasotec (2.5 mg) for high blood pressure; aspirin (81 mg); and Mevacor (lovastatin, 20 mg) for high blood cholesterol.

His exercise tolerance has improved to where he can walk a mile on level ground at a moderate pace without angina. He usually has chest pain only with aggravation and not with exercise. He has dropped from Class III functional capacity to Class I and is now able to engage in activity without pain. He has done extremely well with our therapy and we hope to do more for him.

SIX CASE HISTORIES USING DIET, SUPPLEMENTS, AND CHELATION THERAPY

The last six case histories are examples of people with heart disease that was initially resistant to treatment. To be successful in such cases, it is often necessary to utilize chelation therapy and stress-reduction techniques, and to temporarily continue the use of prescription medications.

Case 20: Stress, an Aggressive Personality, and a Risky Cholesterol Profile Reversed

D.F. was a sixty-eight-year-old male, height 6'2", weight 201 pounds, with a long-standing medical history of coronary artery disease with triple vessel disease (numerous blockages in different areas), and mild left ventricular dysfunction. When walking, he would often experience shortness of breath and chest discomfort. He had cardiac catheterization and a stress thallium test, which were markedly abnormal. His EKG showed wave abnormalities. His total cholesterol was 230, and his HDLs were dangerously low at 28. His medications included Cardizem CD (300 mg); Isordil (isosorbide, 10 mg); Mevacor (20 mg); as well as multiple vitamins. His physical exam was normal, his pulse was regular at 56, and his blood pressure was 118/82. In addition, he had an overly aggressive personality and temporal lobe dysfunction as indicated with BEAM brain mapping.

He agreed to take a low dose of Dilantin (100 mg), use biofeedback and CES, and follow a supplement plan that included: zero-flush niacin (400 mg); 4 capsules fish oil (500 mg); borage oil (4 g); CoQ$_{10}$ (30 mg); carnitine (1 g); zinc (50 mg); N-acetyl-cysteine (500 mg). The following formulas were also prescribed: Heart Formula (#1); Antioxidant Formula (#2); Calcium Formula (#3); Magnesium Formula (#4); and Multivitamin Formula (#9).

After sixty-nine chelation treatments, we confirmed an increase in blood flow in the heart with a PET scan. His overall symptoms when walking had greatly diminished, and he is now able to do more exercise. He underwent biofeedback for stress relaxation for his aggressive personality. Notably, he had an astonishingly low level of LDL cholesterol at 67. His total cholesterol was 147, with an HDL of 38. He feels extremely well and is symptom-free today.

Case 21: Peripheral Vascular Disease (and Other Serious Health Problems) Solved

P.H. was a sixty-four-year-old woman who needed treatment for peripheral vascular disease. She had a history of manic-depressive disorder, general anxiety, and a dependent and histrionic personality. She suffered from cataracts, elevated cholesterol, high blood pressure, hypothyroidism, arthritis, insomnia, was postmenopausal and allergic to various grains. An electrocardiogram showed conduction disturbances. BEAM brain mapping revealed abnormal brain rhythms and other multiple lobe abnormalities. Her exam also indicated weak pulse in the legs and feet (left greater than right), multiple varicosities, hair loss, and skin color changes. The patient refused to go on the proper medications.

P.H. agreed to participate in a complete nutrient program, however. Among her daily supplements: zero-flush niacin (400 mg); Heart Formula (#1); Antioxidant Formula (#2); Multivitamin Formula (#9); fish oil (2 g); and borage oil (3 g). Her medications included Tranxene SD (clorazepate, 22.5 mg) for anxiety, which she refused to go off; natural estrogen and progesterone; Mellaril (thioridazine, 10 mg) for anxiety at different times, as well as Synthroid (levothyroxine) for low thyroid levels; Wellbutrin (bupropion) for depression; Ismo and nitroglycerin for angina; Cardizem for high blood pressure, and Mevacor for elevated cholesterol.

P.H. underwent twenty-two chelation treatments with great success. She had significant improvement of her cramping due to the peripheral vascular disease. She has had successful treatment of her thyroid problems. Her total cholesterol fell from 240 to 199. We have been following her kidney function and adjusting her chelation dose accordingly. She is now symptom-free except for mild cramping in the legs.

Case 22: Symptom Relief from Severe Heart and Vascular Diseases

D.B., a seventy-seven-year-old man, came into the office with subclavian steal syndrome (decreased blood supply to the back of the brain), a reduced opening in the valve of the aorta, and as a result, abnormal flow of blood from the aorta. He also suffered from coronary artery disease. He had generalized anxiety, mild depression, and an aggressive personality. Results from brain mapping showed abnormalities indicative of a temporal lobe disorder. Other health problems included hypothyroidism, benign prostatic hypertrophy (BPH), anemia, irritable bowel syndrome (IBS), and premature ejaculation.

He was taking low doses of Tofranil (imipramine, 50 mg); Klonopin (clonazepam 0.5 mg, at bedtime) for anxiety; Tenormin (atenolol, 50 mg), and Cardizem CD (120 mg) once a day. His EKG was normal. Cardiac catherization showed significant blockages in two main heart vessels (right coronary and left anterior descending) and in the smaller vessel. Bruits (murmurs) in the carotid and subclavian arteries were also discovered.

His daily regimen consisted of six capsules of fish oil (500 mg, A.M. and P.M.); safflower oil (3 tablespoons); Heart Formula (#1); Antioxidant Formula (#2); Magnesium Formula (#4); Multivitamin formula (#9); Brain-Energy Formula (#10); Vitamin C Formula (#14); DHEA (100 mg); Armour desiccated liver (2 g); carnitine (1 g); zero-flush niacin (400 mg); vitamin A (8,500 IU); N-acetyl-cysteine (500 mg); and CoQ_{10} (30 mg). He was tapered off Tofranil and Tenormin. His medications included Xanax (alprazolam, 0.5 mg) to replace Klonopin for anxiety; Ismo (20 mg); testosterone (100 mg/ml); and Cardizem CD (120 mg). He is gradually being weaned off these drugs and is following the Rainbow Diet.

During the course of his chelation therapy, he experienced tremendous symptom relief and a decrease in his cholesterol. His HDL levels rose from 51 to 70. His elevated liver enzymes, which are probably the result of drinking, had normalized. His weight, originally 145 pounds, is now up to 160 pounds. His episodes of depression are now relieved.

Case 23: Circumvention of a Second Bypass

P.B. was a sixty-eight-year-old man with angina. He had already had one bypass, and was headed for another, which he did not think he could go through again. He had an abnormal stress thallium test, which monitors the heart when exercising. The PET scan revealed severe blockage in the left anterior descending artery, and mild to moderate blockage in the right coronary and in the left circumflex arteries. He had anginal pain. Other than a mildly enlarged prostate, his physical exam was unremarkable. He received a prostate-specific antigen (PSA) test and had his testosterone levels checked. He was in male menopause, had testosterone deficiency, and his PSAs (a protein in the blood that can indicate the presence of cancer in the prostate) were normal. He had an aggressive personality disorder, which was confirmed by his abnormal BEAM brain map.

His treatment included the following supplements: emulsified liquid fish oil; Heart Formula (#1); Antioxidant Formula (#2); Magnesium Formula (#4); Multivitamin Formula (#9); Brain-Energy Formula (#10); and choline (50 mg).

Due to the seriousness of his condition, he was prescribed Cardizem CD (240 mg), Ismo (20 mg), and Mevacor (20 mg). His low testosterone is also being treated when he is able to follow-up and comply with the injection, although he doesn't care much about the quality of his sex life and neither does his wife. He is also receiving a low dose of Dilantin to reduce his type-A drive and is using a CES device and biofeedback.

We treated P.B. with forty-six chelation treatments and with the Ismo and Cardizem. He has had continued weight problems, fluctuating up to 180 pounds, with initial cholesterol of 281. He has been willing to take Mevacor along with the niacin. He has not been willing to follow his diet regimen aggressively. His repeat PET scan to reassess his blockages showed mild blockage in his left circumflex, right coronary, and left anterior descending arteries. Remarkably, his EKG is normal and cholesterol is now controlled. He is symptom-free.

Case 24: In the Best Health Ever

E.S., a sixty-four-year-old male, 240 pounds, presented to us with elevated total cholesterol of 258, high blood pressure, and angina. He had had bypass surgery in the mid-1980s for one blocked vessel. In 1991 E.S. had a second bypass surgery, this time for three blocked arteries. Additional testing found him to have memory loss, low sex drive, a co-dependent personality according to the Millon personality-trait stress test, a brain-map assessment indicative of impending Alzheimerlike symptoms, and a blockage in the carotid arteries.

His medications presently included a low dose of the beta-blocker Tenormin (50 mg); Cardizem CD (240 mg); and Eldepryl (selegiline hydrochloride, 5 mg).

E.S.'s treatment included protocol for benign prostatic hypertrophy (BPH), high blood pressure, brain mapping abnormalities, and angina. Twenty-seven chelation treatments were administered and the following supplement therapy prescribed: 4 capsules fish oil (500 mg); one tablet each of our Antioxidant Formula (#2); Magnesium Formula (#4); Multivitamin Formula (#9); Brain-Energy Formula (#10); Vitamin C Formula (#14); zero-flush niacin (400 mg); choline (50 mg); CoQ_{10} (30 mg); DHEA (100 mg), and N-acetyl-cysteine (500 mg).

E.S. also received treatment with injectable testosterone for low testosterone, which helped him to recover his sex drive. The appetite suppressant Ionamin (phentermine) helped him lose weight and improve his memory; otherwise he is off all medications and control of his high blood pressure significantly improved. He went from a weight of 240 to 215. He says he is in the best health of his life.

Case 25: Complete Reversal of Heart Disease and Peripheral Vascular Disease

C.V. was a seventy-two-year-old woman with hypothyroidism who was diagnosed with breast cancer, high blood pressure, and blockages in the carotid arteries and arteries of her lower extremities.

Despite her refusal to quit smoking (one to five cigarettes a day), C.V. started a regimen that included Nolvadex (tamoxifen); Prozac (fluoxetine) for depression; Deseryl (trazodone, 50–100 mg) for panic attacks; and a wide range of nutrients. Her daily regimen included: borage oil (4 g); Antioxidant Formula (#2); Magnesium Formula (#4); Multivitamin Formula (#9); Brain-Energy Formula (#10); Vitamin C Formula (#14); vitamin A (8,500 IU); and zero-flush niacin (400 mg). In addition, she received testosterone (5 mg); DHEA (100 mg); and Armour desiccated liver for low thyroid (1.5 g).

C.V. was able to completely reverse the blockages in her carotid arteries and arteries in her lower extremities within one year after being identified using the Doppler Test. We were able to hold her breast cancer in check while obtaining complete and successful treatment of her depression and high blood pressure. Chelation therapy was very successful at pulling out excess lead and cadmium for her body. C.V. had a complete reversal of her heart disease by combining all aspects of the program with the nutrients, CES, and in this case, medication.

Success Stories of Heart Failure Patients

Years of high blood pressure and coronary artery disease, with resulting myocardial infarction, can cause chronic strain on the heart, gradually weakening the heart muscle and compromising its ability to pump out blood. The functional capacity of the heart muscle is reflected by its ejection faction (EF), which is measured using an echocardiogram.

Ejection fraction is the fraction of the blood ejected by the heart's left ventricle. Normally, the ejection fraction is about 55 percent. When it goes down, it results in a serious condition known as congestive heart failure. Shortness of breath on exertion, cough, fatigue, cardiac enlargement, leg edema, and at times, enlargement of the liver are manifestations of congestive heart failure.

The following patients came to us with severe congestive heart failure and other cardiovascular abnormalities. Using the No-More Hypertension and Heart Disease Program, each one improved their EKG, their ejection fraction, and their life.

Patient and Symptoms	EF Before Program	EF After Program
P.T., a seventy-eight-year-old male, with severe cardiac failure due to longstanding, uncontrolled high blood pressure. *Time duration:* 1 year later	38%	54%
E.F., a fifty-four-year-old woman, with severe heart failure as a result of extensive damage from myocardial infarction. *Time duration:* 4 years later	20%	45%
K.W., a fifty-seven-year-old woman, went from severe left ventricular dysfunction due to high blood pressure and ischemic heart disease to mild ventricular dysfunction. *Time duration:* 1 year later	25%	45%

Patient and Symptoms	EF Before Program	EF After Program
M.W., a seventy-eight- year old male, with congestive heart failure, high blood pressure, coronary artery disease, and atrial fibrillation (abnormally fast irregular heart rhythm). His echocardiogram showed enlargement of the left side of the heart and abnormalities in three heart valves. *Time duration:* 2.5 years later	38%	54%
S.M, fifty-seven-year old female, with congenital heart disease surgically repaired years ago, left ventricular dysfunction, severe right ventricular dilation, pulmonary hypertension, and other medical problems. *Time duration:* 1.5 years later	50%	60%

As you can see from the case studies, the No-More Hypertension and Heart Disease Program works. From heart palpitations to triple vessel coronary artery disease, from creeping blood pressure to the precipice of an impending bypass—no matter the type or severity of your heart disease—it can be slowed, stopped, and even completely reversed with our program.

The key is to use the full armament available to you. Diet, nutritional supplements, exercise, weight control, and stress reduction are essential, as, in some cases, are hormone therapy, chelation, and the many other therapies you've read about in this book. Remember, the heart is connected to the whole body. Really effective treatment of high blood pressure and heart disease involves restoring health not only to the heart and vascular system, but also to the key organs and body systems—the kidneys, adrenal glands, thyroid, pancreas, sex organs, and brain. It requires a total approach like the No-More Hypertension and Heart Disease Program. Follow this approach and you can become the healthy, heart disease-free human being you were meant to be, and maintain that lowered cardiovascular risk for the rest of your life.

Heart-Healthy Recipes

Here are more than a dozen recipes to complement the eating options presented in Chapter 4. Ingredients marked with an asterisk (*) are considered hypertension-breaking substances as they contribute to lowering blood pressure and/or cholesterol. Don't hesitate to experiment and be creative. In addition, there are many good cookbooks on the market using the wholesome ingredients and common-sense approaches to healthful eating presented in the Rainbow Diet. Check out your local bookstore or library.

Anti-Hypertension Shake #1

*This delicious shake is for hypertensives
who want to restrict their carbohydrate intake.*

YIELD: 1 SERVING

3 ¼ cups crushed ice

2–3 tablespoons safflower oil* (as directed by physician)

½ banana*

1 tablespoon freshly ground flaxseed* (for fiber)

Sweetener such as Stevia to taste

Dash of non-alcoholic fruit or vanilla extract

Nutmeg or cinnamon to taste

1. In a blender or food processor, combine all ingredients and whip until smooth.

Variation: Substitute ²/₃ cups fresh fruit* for the banana* (preferably melon or apple). Use 3–4 ice cubes instead of the crushed ice.

Anti-Hypertension Shake #2

A protein-packed fruit smoothie high in complex carbohydrates.

YIELD: 1 SERVING

1 package soft tofu*, drained

1½ cups any fresh or frozen fruit* such as bananas,
berries, cherries, papayas

1 tablespoon freshly ground flaxseed* (for fiber)

Sweetener such as Stevia to taste

Spice of your choice to taste—such as cinnamon,
nutmeg, lemon juice, vanilla

Bottled water or low fat, skim, rice, or soy* milk,
if needed, to desired consistency.

1. In a blender or food processor, combine all ingredients and whip until smooth.

Variation 1: To make a vegetable version of this shake, omit sweetener and spices and substitute any hypertension-breaking vegetable*. Add 1 teaspoon of olive oil* and salt substitute to taste.

Variation 2: For a super hypertension and cholesterol-breaking shake, add 2–3 tablespoons of safflower oil.*

Anti-Hypertension Shake #3

A rich, velvety drink for hypertensives with normal weight.

YIELD: 1 SERVING

2–3 tablespoons safflower oil*
(as directed by physician)

1 small to medium banana

1 tablespoon freshly ground flaxseeds* for fiber

5 ounces low fat, skim, rice or soy* milk

Sweetener such as Stevia to taste

Orange zest or fresh grated ginger to taste

1. In a blender or food processor, combine all ingredients and whip until smooth.

Variation: Use only 4 ounces milk or milk alternative and
½ banana. Add 3–4 ice cubes and a dash of non-alcoholic fruit
or vanilla extract.

Anti-Hypertension Lemonade

YIELD: 1 SERVING

7 teaspoons freshly squeezed lemon or lime juice

8 ounces no-salt seltzer

Sweetener such as Stevia to taste

1. Combine all ingredients in a glass and stir well.

CONDIMENTS AND SPREADS

Healthy Heart Spread

*Don't we all love to dip and nibble? This delicious sauce is
wonderful as a pita bread filling, spread, or cracker dip.*

YIELD: 4 SERVINGS

1 medium eggplant, peeled and sliced
into ½" thick rounds

1 small onion*, finely chopped or grated

3 tablespoons sugar-free, salt-free
safflower oil mayonnaise*

Tabasco and low-sodium tamari or
soy sauce with ginger to taste

1. Place eggplant slices on an ungreased baking sheet.

2. Bake at 375°F for approximately 30 minutes.

3. Dice and puree by hand or in blender or a food processor
until smooth.

4. Fold in onion, mayonnaise, and Tabasco.

Variation: Add 1–2 cloves garlic, mashed or minced or one fresh
tomato, finely chopped.

Jicama-Chili Pepper Relish

This jazzy, colorful dish combines the mild sweet flavor of jicama (a root vegetable pronounced "KEE-k-ma"), carrots and zucchini, with spicy peppers in a rich, slightly smoky-tasting relish with jolt.

YIELD: 4 SERVINGS

1 medium jicama (about 1 pound), peeled and cut into $\frac{1}{2}$ inch cubes*

1 large carrot, peeled*

1 medium zucchini, scrubbed and trimmed*

1–2 pickled chipotle peppers in adobo sauce, with liquid*

1 cup finely chopped onion*

4 garlic cloves, peeled and minced*

1 bay leaf

6 whole black peppercorns

$\frac{1}{2}$ cup water

$\frac{1}{3}$ cup olive oil*

1 tablespoon chopped cilantro or parsley*

1 teaspoon dried oregano

Vinegar to taste

Low fat yogurt to taste

1. Using a knife, remove skin from jicama. Cut into half-inch dice. Place jicama pieces in a bowl.

2. Lightly steam carrot until cooked. Cut into half-inch dice. Add to the bowl with jicama. Lightly steam zucchini. Dice into half-inch cubes. Add to the bowl.

3. Drain the chipotles, reserving the pickling sauce (one chili makes a relatively mild marinade; use 2 if desired). Cut chilies open lengthwise, scrape out the seeds. Finely chop, and place in a separate, medium-sized bowl.

4. Add onion, garlic, bay leaf, peppercorns, vinegar, water, olive oil, and cilantro or parsley to chipotles in bowl. Blend in the reserved chipotle sauce. Crumble oregano and add to bowl. Whisk all the ingredients together and pour the marinade over jicama mixture. Toss vegetables with the marinade to coat completely.

5. Put in a non-reactive kettle or soup pot. Bring to a boil. Cook 10–12 minutes until tender. Drain.

6. Return vegetables to pan, add yogurt and oil.

7. Mash ingredients until coarse. Blend thoroughly and serve warm.

SIDE DISHES

Potato and Parsnip Puree

Here's a twist on classic mashed potatoes but without the fat and high-starch content. Parsnips are rich in complex carbohydrates and have the melt-in-your-mouth richness everyone loves.

YIELD: 4 SERVINGS

1½ pounds russet potatoes, about 4 medium potatoes (approx. 3 cups)

2 large parsnips*, trimmed and scraped, sliced crosswise (approx. 2 cups)*

1 large yellow onion, peeled and sliced*

2 garlic cloves, peeled and minced*

Salt substitute to taste

½ cup low-fat yogurt*

1 teaspoon of olive oil*

½ cup chives (or other herb of your choice)

Pinch of nutmeg

Freshly ground pepper to taste

1. Peel and quarter potatoes. Combine potatoes with parsnips, onion, and garlic in large saucepan. Add water to cover, add salt substitute, and bring to a boil.

2. Cook 10–12 minutes until tender. Drain.

3. Return vegetables to saucepan. Add yogurt and oil.

4. Mash ingredients until coarse. Add remaining seasonings, blend thoroughly and serve warm.

Variation: Substitute carrots or celery root for parsnips; use Jerusalem artichokes in place of potatoes to reduce starch.

MAIN DISHES

Two-Herb Pesto

You can put this traditionally high-fat, high-sodium sauce back on the menu. Asiago (similar to Parmesan) has 75 percent less fat than conventional grating cheeses.

YIELD: 4 SERVINGS

8 walnuts (shelled)

¼ cup grated Asiago* or low fat Parmesan cheese*

2 cloves crushed garlic*

½ cup olive oil

1 ½ cups fresh chopped parsley*, stems included

½ cup fresh chopped basil, stems included*

1–2 tablespoons boiling water

Tabasco sauce or potassium salt substitute to taste*

1. Put nuts, cheese, and garlic in blender or food processor. With blender running, add oil in a thin stream, blending until mixture is smooth. Add herbs, a few sprigs at a time.

2. With blender still running, add boiling water to bring mixture to a mayonnaiselike consistency.

3. Season with tabasco sauce or salt substitute. Serve over wholewheat or low-carbohydrate soy pasta, or spread on cooked fish.

Chinese Steamed-Fish Kebabs with Almonds

Chunks of succulent fatty fish essential for keeping blood pressure on an even keel and for boosting levels of good cholesterol make this an exceptionally heart-healthy dish.

YIELD: 2 SERVINGS

12 ounces snapper*, salmon* or halibut* steaks, ¾-inch thick

2 teaspoons of low-sodium tamari or soy sauce

1 teaspoon lemon juice

1 teaspoon safflower* or olive oil*

1 clove garlic*, minced

⅛ teaspoon red pepper flakes*

2 scallions* with tops, cut into 1-inch strips

2 teaspoons thinly sliced almonds*

2 tablespoons of minced cilantro (Chinese parsley)*

1. Rinse fish; pat dry. Cut into serving portions; set aside.

2. Combine next five ingredients through red pepper in a small bowl; set aside.

3. Boil water in bottom half of steamer, or any deep saucepan or electric skillet with a tight-fitting lid. Arrange fish on top rack of steamer; brush with soy sauce mixture, and scatter scallions on top. Cover and steam 5 to 6 minutes until fish is opaque.

4. Using a spatula, transfer fish to serving platter. Sprinkle with almonds and garnish with cilantro.

Salmon Kebabs

Leftovers make tasty salads for lunch. If you have a wheat allergy, use wheat-free tamari sauce called shoyu, available at natural food stores.

YIELD: 2 TO 3 GENEROUS SERVINGS

1 pound fresh wild Alaskan salmon* or any firm-flesh fish, cut into 1" by 1" squares

2 tablespoons chopped garlic*

1 tablespoon chopped ginger root*

1 cup safflower oil*

½ cup low-sodium tamari or soy sauce

8 cherry tomatoes*

1 small onion* cut into quarters

1. Dice salmon and place in a bowl. Make a marinade with garlic, ginger root, and safflower oil and coat fish pieces well. Marinate for 15–30 minutes.

2. Drain and alternate salmon, tomato, onion on skewers.

3. Cook on hot outdoor grill or indoor hibachi, approximately 5 minutes on each side.

Variation: Leave fish in steak form and marinate. Grill 7–10 minutes on each side.

SALADS AND SALAD DRESSINGS

Two-Way Total Health Salad

Chock full of herbs and high-quality protein, these light, delicious, and easily prepared salads can quickly become a main course for a meal.

YIELD: 6 TO 8 SERVINGS

Salad Base

¼ cup safflower* or extra-virgin olive oil*

2 tablespoons herb vinegar

⅓ cup green onions*, thinly sliced

2 garlic cloves*, crushed and diced

Pepper

Salt substitute to taste

Salad Option #1 with Herbs

¼ cup fresh parsley*, finely minced

¼ cup fresh tarragon*, finely minced

1 tablespoon fresh dill*, minced

1 tablespoon celery leaves*, minced

½ pound green snap beans, lightly steamed and cooled, in 1-inch lengths

2 hard-boiled eggs, coarsely chopped

Salad Option #2 with Seafood

¼ cup fresh basil*, finely chopped

¼ cup fresh chervil*, finely chopped

½ cup fresh celery*, finely diced

1-1½ cups cooked salmon, mackerel or trout* in bite-sized chunks

3 cups mixed salad greens*

1. Combine salad base ingredients. Whisk oil together with vinegar, garlic, salt substitute, and pepper.

2. Assemble ingredients for salad option #1 or #2, and mix well.

3. Combine salad base ingredients with salad option ingredients. Marinate at least thirty minutes before serving.

Tangy Cucumber Dressing

An all-purpose, low-sodium, high-potassium dressing
and a perfect complement to the tanginess of mustard greens,
cabbage, fresh spinach, and tender greens.

YIELD: 1 CUP

1 12-ounce cucumber, pared, seeded,
and coarsely chopped*

½ cup parsley sprigs*

¼ cup plain nonfat yogurt

1 sliced scallion* with top

1 tablespoon tarragon vinegar

1 tablespoon Dijon-style mustard

1 clove sliced garlic*

½ teaspoon celery seed

½ teaspoon dried dill weed*

Few drops Worcestershire sauce

1. Place all ingredients in blender and process until smooth.

2. Refrigerate several hours to blend flavors. May be used as a dip for vegetables or crackers. Refrigerated, keeps one week.

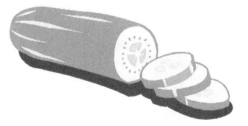

APPENDIX B

Dr. Braverman's Special Formulas

Although the following formulas have been used to successfully treat thousands of cases of high blood pressure and heart disease, you may choose to substitute another brand. Just be sure that the product you choose contains the same quality ingredients; if several ingredients are missing you may need to supplement these individually. You'll find that all formulas vary in the types and amounts of ingredients they contain. So, you'll need to do some calculating to get the right dosage for the equivalent daily amount if using other supplements. If you opt to use our formulas, they can be purchased online at www.pathmed.com, www.totalhealthsupplements.com, or www.edgeeffect.org, or by calling (888) 231-PATH or (212) 213-6155.

DR. BRAVERMAN'S SPECIAL FORMULAS			
PRODUCT	AMOUNT	PRODUCT	AMOUNT
HEART FORMULA #1			
Garlic powder (odorless)	200 mg	Chromium (chloride)	26.7 mcg
Taurine	200 mg	Niacinamide	50 mg
Magnesium (oxide)	50 mg	Vitamin C (ascorbic acid)	40 mg
Potassium (chloride)	6.7 mg	Molybdenum (chelate)	40 mcg
Selenium (sodium sel.)	20 mcg	Vitamin B_6	50 mg
Zinc (chelate)	4 mg	Beta-carotene	1,222 IU
ANTIOXIDANT FORMULA #2			
Vitamin A (beta-carotene)	8,500 IU	L-cysteine	250 mg
Vitamin C (ascorbic acid)	250 mg	Selenium (selenomethionine)	50 mcg
Vitamin E	100 IU	Niacinamide	10 mg

DR. BRAVERMAN'S SPECIAL FORMULAS (cont.)			
PRODUCT	**AMOUNT**	**PRODUCT**	**AMOUNT**
CALCIUM FORMULA #3			
Calcium (citrate)	270 mg	Boron	0.5 mg
Manganese (chelate)	1.5 mg	Strontium	0.5 mg
Vitamin D_3	135 IU		
MAGNESIUM FORMULA #4			
Vitamin B_6	65 mg	Zinc (chelate)	15 mg
Magnesium (oxide)	470 mg		
MULTIVITAMIN AND MINERAL FORMULA #9			
Vitamin A (beta-carotene)	1,000 IU	Biotin	50 mcg
Vitamin C (ascorbic acid)	200 mg	Pantothenic acid	6 mg
Vitamin D	200 IU	Calcium (carbonate)	15 mg
Vitamin E	20 mg	Iron (chelate)	5 mg
Thiamine	5 mg	Iodine (kelp)	100 mcg
Riboflavin	5 mg	Magnesium (oxide)	12 mg
Niacin/niacinamide	15 mg	Molybdenum (chelate)	12 mg
Vitamin B_6	5 mg	Manganese (chelate)	1 mg
Folate	125 mcg	GTF chromium (polynicotinate)	60 mcg
Vitamin B_{12}	60 mcg	Zinc (chelate)	5 mg
BRAIN-ENERGY FORMULA #10			
DL-Phenylalanine	300 mg	Octacosanol	2 mg
L-Tyrosine	200 mg	Rhodiola Rosea Root extract	75 mg
DL-Methionine	60 mg		
ZINC FORMULA #13			
Iodine (kelp)	30 mcg	Molybdenum	130 mcg
Zinc (gluconate)	20 mg	Vanadium	30 mcg
Manganese (chelate)	1 mg	Rubidium	30 mcg
Boron	130 mcg		
VITAMIN C FORMULA #14			
Vitamin C (ascorbic acid)	160 mg	Bioflavonoids	65 mg
Niacinamide	10 mg	DL-Methionine	65 mg
Quercetin	130 mg		

Recommended Reading

Atkins, Robert. *Dr. Atkins' New Diet Revolution* (2nd edition). New York, NY: M. Evans & Company, Inc., 2002.

Braverman, Eric. *The PATH Wellness Manual* (2nd edition). Skillman, NJ: Publications for Achieving Total Health, 1995.

Moore, Thomas. *The Dash Diet for Hypertension.* New York, NY: Simon & Schuster, 2002.

Ornish, Dean. *Dr. Dean Ornish's Program for Reversing Heart Disease* (2nd edition). New York, NY: Ballantine Books, 1996.

Sinatra, Stephen and Sinatra, Jan. *Lower Your Blood Pressure in Eight Weeks.* New York, NY: Ballantine Books, 2003.

References

Chapter 1

Daly, J., Sindone, A.P., Thompson, D.R., et al. "Barriers to participation in and adherence to cardiac rehabilitation programs: a critical literature review." *Prog Cardiovasc Nurs.* 2002 Winter;17(1):8–17.

Dosh, S.A. "The treatment of adults with essential hypertension." *J Fam Pract.* 2002 Jan;51(1):74–80.

Falk, E., Zhon, J., Moller, J. "Homocysteine and atherothrombosis." *Lipids.* 2001;36 Suppl:S3–11.

Freeman, L.M., Rush, J.E., Cahalane, A.K., et al. "Dietary pattern of dogs with cardiac disease." *J Nutr.* 2002 Jun;132(6 Suppl 2):1632S–3S.

Kannel, W.B., Castelli, W.P., Gordon, T., et al. "Serum cholesterol, lipoproteins, and the risk of coronary heart disease; the Framingham Study." *Annals of Internal Medicine.* 1971;74:1–12.

Markovitz, J., et al., "Psychological predictors of hypertension in the Framingham Study." *JAMA.* 1993;370:20,2439–42.

McKee, M., Perry, J. "Ischaemic heart disease—more than just lipids." *Eur J Public Health.* 2002 Dec;12(4):241–2. No abstracts available.

Pickering, T. "Tension and hypertension." *JAMA.* 1993;370:20,2494.

Rao, S. "Nutritional status of the Indian population." *J Biosci.* 2001 Nov;26(4 Suppl): 481–9.

Ravnskov, U. "Diet-heart disease hypothesis is wishful thinking." *BMJ.* 2002 Jan 26;324(7331):238.

Rosick, R. "The new guidelines for hypertension." *Life Extension.* 2004; (collector's edition):91–98.

Sanchez-Muniz, F.J., Merinero, M.C., Rodriguez-Gil, S., et al. "Dietary fat saturation affects apolipoprotein AII levels and HDL composition in post-menopausal women." *J Nutr.* 2002 Jan;132(1):50–4.

Schulpis, K.H., Karikas, G.A., Papakonstantinou, E. "Homocysteine and other vascular risk factors in patients with phenylketonuria on a diet." *Acta Paodiatr.* 2002;91(8):905–9.

Sempos, C.T. "Do body iron stores increase the risk of developing coronary heart disease?" *Am J Clin Nutr.* 2002 Sep;76(3):501–3.

SoRelle, R. "One in 5 at risk for congestive heart failure." *Circulation.* 2002 Dec 10; 106(24):e9066–7.

Taha, D. "Hyperlipidemia in children with type 2 diabetes mellitus." *J Pediatr Endocrinol Metab.* 2002 Apr;15 Suppl 1:505–7.

Volozh, O., Solodkaya, E., Abina, J., et al. "Some biological cardiovascular risk factors and diet in samples of the male population of Tallinn, Estonia in 1984/1985 and 1992/1993." *Eur J Public Health.* 2002 Mar;12(1):16–21.

Wong, N.D., Pio, J., Valencia,R., et al. "Distribution of C-reactive protein and its relation to risk factors and coronary heart disease risk estimation in the National Health and Nutrition Examination Survey (NHANES) III." *Prev Cardiol.* 2001 Summer;4(3):109–114.

Chapter 2

"Heart disease prevention." *AIDS Treat News.* 2001 Jan 25;(377):2–3.

Halm, M.A., Denker, J. "Primary Prevention Programs to Reduce Heart Disease Risk in Women." *Clin Nurse Spec.* 2003 Mar;17(2):101–109.

Khosh F., Khosh, M. "Natural approach to hypertension." *Altern Med Rev.* 2001 Dec;6(6):590–600.

Messinger-Rapport, B.J., Sprecher, D. "Prevention of cardiovascular diseases. Coronary artery disease, congestive heart failure, and stroke." *Clin Geriatr Med.* 2002 Aug;18 (3):463–83, vii.

National Institutes of Health/National Heart, Lung, and Blood Institute. "The Sixth Report of the Joint National Committee on Prevention, Detection, Evaluation and Treatment of High Blood Pressure." Bethesda, MD: NIH, 1997 (NIH publication no. 98–4080s).

Nordoy, A. "Statins and omega-3 fatty acids in the treatment of dyslipidemia and coronary heart disease." *Minerva Med.* 2002 Oct;93(5): 357–63.

Slama, M., Susie, D., Frohlich, E.D. "Prevention of hypertension." *Curr Opin Cardiol.* 2002 Sep;17(5):531–6.

Chapter 4

Caramia, G. "Polyunsaturated fatty acids; omega-3 in child development." *Pediatr Med Chir.* 2002 Sep-Oct;24(5):337–45.

Courts, A. "Nutrition and the life cycle 4: the healthy diet for the adult." *Br J Nurs.* 2001 Mar 22–April 11;10(6):362:364–9.

Daniels, L. "Diet and coronary heart disease: advice on a cardioprotective diet." *Br J Community Nurs.* 2002 Jul;7(7):346–50.

DASH Collaborative Research Group. "The effect of dietary patterns on blood pressure: results from the Dietary Approaches to Stop Hypertension (DASH) clinical trial. *Current Concepts in Hyptertension.* 1998 Nov;2:4–5.

DeLorgeril, M., Salen, P. "Fish and N-3 fatty acids for the prevention and treatment of coronary heart disease: nutrition is not pharmacology." *Am J Med.* 2002 Mar;112(4):316–9.

Hernandez-Diaz, S., Marinez-Losa, E., Fernandex-Jarne, F., et al. "Dietary folate and the risk of nonfatal myocardial infarction." *Epidemiology.* 2002 Nov;13(6):700–6.

Jenkins, D.J., Kendall, C.W., Jackson, C.J., et al. "Effects of high- and low-isoflavone soyfoods on blood lipids, oxidized LDL, homocysteine, and blood pressure in hyperlipidemic men and women. *Am J Clin Nutr.* 2002 Aug; 76 (2):365–72.

John, J.H., Ziebland, S., Yudkin, P., et al. "Effects of fruit and vegetable consumption on plasma antioxidant concentrations and blood pressure: a randomised controlled trial." *Lancet.* 2002 Jun 8;359(9322):1969–74.

Joshipura, K., Ascherio, A., Manson, J., Stampfer, M. et al. "Fruit and vegetable intake in relation to risk of ischemic stroke." *JAMA.* Oct 6, 1999; 2821(13):1233.

Kernan-Schroeder, D., Cunningham, M. "Glycemic control and beyond: the ABCs of standards of care for type 2 diabetes and cardiovascular disease." *J Cardiovasc Nurs.* 2002 Jan;16(2):44–54.

Liu, S., Manson, J.E., Buring, J.E., et al. "Relation between a diet with a high glycemic load and plasma concentrations of high-sensitivity C-reactive protein in middle-aged women." *Am J Clin Nutr.* 2002 Mar;75(3):492–8.

Luippold, G., Zimmermann, C., Mai, M., et al. "Dopamine D(3) receptors and salt-dependent hypertension. *J Am Soc Nephrol.* 2001 Nov;12(11): 2272–9.

Maddox, D.A., Alavi, F.K., Silbernick, E.M., Zawada, E.T. "Protective effects of a soy diet in preventing obesity-linked renal disease." *Kidney Int.* 2002 Jan;61(1):96–104.

Mann, J.I. "Diet and risk of coronary heart disease and type 2 diabetes." *Lancet.* 2002 Sep 7;360(9335):783–9.

Miller, E.C., Giovannucci, B., Erdman, J.W., et al. "Tomato products, lycopene, and prostate cancer risk." *Urol Clin North Am.* 2002 Feb;29(1): 80–93.

Nakamura, T., Azuma, A., Kuribayashi, T., et al. "Serum fatty acid levels, dietary style and coronary heart disease in three neighbouring areas in Japan: the Kumihama study." *Br J Nutr.* 2003 Feb;89(2):267–72.

Nappo, F., Loreto, M., Giugliano, G., et al. "Elevated plasma free fatty acid concentrations do not modify cardiac repolarization in patients treated by electrolyte-glucose-insulin infusion." *J Endocrinol Invest.* 2002 Jul–Aug; 25(7):RC19–22.

Ness, A.R. "Is olive oil a key ingredient in the Mediterranean recipe for health?" *Int J Epidemiol.* 2002 Apr;31(2):481–2.

Ness, A.R., Gallacher, J.E., Bennett, P.D., et al. "Advice to eat fish and mood: a randomized controlled trial in men with angina." *Nutr Neurosci.* 2003 Feb;6 (1):63–5.

Nordoy, A., Marchioli, R., Arnesen, H., et al. "n-3 polyunsaturated fatty acids and cardiovascular diseases." *Lipids.* 2002;36 Suppl:S127–9.

Owen, R.W., Giacosa, A., Hull, W.E., et al. "Olive-oil consumption and health: the possible role of antioxidants." *Lancet Oncol.* 2000 Oct;1: 107–12.

Patient information. "Soybeans: good for your heart." *Adv Nurse Pract.* 2002 May; 10(5):85.

Pereira, M.A., Jacobs, D.R., Pins, J.J., et al. "Effect of whole grains on insulin sensitivity in overweight hyperinsulinemic adults." *Am J Clin Nutr.* 2002 May;75(5):848–55.

Perez-Jimenez, F., Lopez-Miranda, J., Mata, P. "Protective effect of dietary monounsaturated fat on arteriosclerosis: beyond cholesterol." *Atherosclerosis.* 2002 Aug;163(2):385–98.

Pickering, T.G. "Diet wars: from Atkins to the Zone. Who is right?" *J Clin Hypertens* (Greenwich). 2002 Mar-Apr;4(2):130–3.

Quies, J.L., Aguilera, C., Mesa, M.D., et al. "An ethanolic-aqueous extract of Curcuma longa decreases the susceptibility of liver microsomes and mitochondria to lipid peroxidation in atherosclerotic rabbits. *Biofactors.* 1998;8(1–2):51–7.

Quiles, J.L., Mesa, M.D., Ramirez-Tortosa, M.C., et al. "Curcuma longa extract supplementation reduces oxidative stress and attenuates aortic fatty acid streak development in rabbits. *Arterioscler Thromb Vasc Biol.* 2002 Jul 1;22(7):1225–31.

Ramirez-Tortosa, M.C., Mesa, M.D., Aguilera, M.C., et al. "Oral administration of a turmeric extract inhibits LDL oxidation and has hypocholesterolemic effects in rabbits with experimental atherosclerosis. *Atherosclerosis.* Dec 1999;147(2):371–8.

Rao, A.V. "Lycopene, tomatoes, and the prevention of coronary heart disease." *Exp Biol Med* (Maywood). 2002 Nov;227(10):908–13.

Rizkalla, S.W., Bellisle, F., Slama, G. "Health benefits of low-glycemic index foods, such as pulses, in diabetic patients and healthy individuals." *Br J Nutr.* 2002 Dec;88 Suppl 3:S255–62.

Rosenberg, J.H. "Fish—food to calm the heart." *N Engl J Med.* 2002 Apr 11;346(15):1102–3.

Sharma, A.M., et al. "Effect of Dietary Salt Restriction on Urinary Serotonin and 5-Hydroxyindoleacetic Acid Execretion." *Man, Journal of Hypertension.* 1993;11:1381–86.

Singh, R.B., Dubnov, G., Niaz, M.A., et al. "Effect of an Indo-Mediterranean diet on progression of coronary artery disease in high risk patients

(Indo-Mediterranean Diet Heart Study): a randomized single-blind trial." *Lancet.* 2002 Nov 9;360(9344):1455–61.

Stark, A.H., Madar, Z. "Olive oil as a functional food: epidemiology and nutritional approaches." *Nutr Rev.* 2002 Jun;60(6):170–6.

Wolk, A., Manson, J., Stampfer, M., et al. "Long-term intake of dietary fiber and decreased risk of coronary heart disease among women." *JAMA.* June 2, 1999;281 (21):1998.

Knekt, P., Jarvinen, R., Reunanen, A., et al. "Flavonoid intake and coronary mortality in Finland: a cohort study. *BMJ.* 1996;312(7029):478–81.

Chapter 5

Braverman, E. and Weissberg, E. "Nutritional Treatments for Hypertension." *Journal of Orthomolecular Medicine.* 1992;7(4):221–24.

Cho, K.H., Eim, E.S., Chen, J.D. "Taurine intake and excretion in patients undergoing long term enteral nutrition." *Adv Exp Med Biol.* 2000;483: 605–12.

Duffy, S.J., Gokce, N., Holbrook, M., et al. "Treatment of hypertension with ascorbic acid." *Lancet.* 1999;354(9195):2048–49.

Hardy, D.B. "n-3 fatty acids and the risk of sudden death." *N Engl J Med.* 2002 Aug 15;347(7):531–3.

Jacob, R.A., Sotoudein, G. "Vitamin C function and status in chronic disease." *Nutr Clin Care.* 2002 Mar–Apr;5(2):66–74.

Jialal, I., Traber, M., Deveraj, S. "Is there a vitamin E paradox?" *Current Opinion in Lipidology,* 2001;12:49–53.

Kumar, K.V. and Das, U.N. "Are free radicals involved in the pathology of human essential hypertension? *Free Rad Res Commun.* 1993;19(1):59–66.

Marchioli, R., Schweiger, C., Tavazzi, L., et al. "Efficacy of n-3 polyunsaturated fatty acids after myocardial infarction: results of GISSI-Prevenzione trial. Gruppo Italiano per lo Studio della Sopravvivenza nell'Infarto Miocardico." *Lipids.* 2001;36 Suppl:S119–26.

Mennen, L.I., deCourey, G.P., Guilland, J.C., et al. "Homocysteine, cardiovascular disease risk factors, and habitual diet in the French Supplementation with Antioxidant Vitamins and Minerals Study." *Am J Clin Nutr.* 2002 Dec; 76(6):1279–89.

Plotnick, G.D., Corretti, M.C., Vogel, R.A. "Effect of antioxidant vitamins on the transient impairment of endothelium-dependent brachial artery vasoactivity following a single high-fat meal. *JAMA.* 1997;278:1682–86.

Preuss, H.G., Clouatre, D., Mohamadi, A., et al. "Wild garlic has a greater effect than regular garlic on blood pressure and blood chemistries in rats." *Int Urol Nephrol.* 2001;32(4):525–30.

Mela, T., Galvin, J.M., McGovern, B.A. "Magnesium deficiency during lactation as a precipitant of ventricular tachyarrhythmias." *Pacing Clin Electrophysiol.* 2002 Feb;25 (2):231–3.

Rosick, R. "The new guidelines for hypertension." *Life Extension.* 2004; (collector's edition):91–98.

Schectman, G. J. Hiatt. "Dose-response characteristics of cholesterol-lowering drug therapies." *Ann Intern Med.* 1996 Dec; 125(12):990–1000.

Silagy, C.A. and Neil, H.A. "A meta-analysis of the effect of garlic on blood pressure." *J Hypertens.* 1994 Apr;12(4):463–68.

Stephens, N.G., Parsons, A., Schofield, P.M., et al. "Randomized controlled trial of vitamin E in patients with coronary disease: Cambridge Heart Antioxidant Study (CHAOS). *Lancet.* 1996;347: 781–86.

Teo, K., et al. "Effect of intravenous magnesium on mortality in myocardial infarction." *Circulation.* 1990;82:111–39.

Toft, I. Bonaa, K.H., Ingebretsen, O.C., et al. "Effects of n-3 polyunsaturated fatty acids on glucose homeostasis and blood pressure in essential hypertension." *Ann Intern Med.* 1995 Dec 15;123(12):911–18.

Venbo, B., Voutilainen, S., Valkonen, V.P., et al. "Arginine intake, blood pressure, and the incidence of acute coronary events in men: the Kuopio Ischaemic Heart Disease Risk Factor Study." *Am J Clin Nutr.* 2002 Aug;76 (2):359–64.

Witteman, J.C., Wilett, W.C., Stampfer, M.J., et al. "A prospective study of nutritional factors and hypertension among U.S. women." *Circulation.* 1989 Nov;80(5):1320–27.

Yokoyama, T., Date, C., Kokubo, Y., et al. "Serum vitamin C concentration was inversely associated with subsequent 20-year incidence of stroke in a Japanese rural community: the Shibata study." *Stroke.* 2000;31(10): 2287–94.

Duffy, S.J., Gokce, N., Holbrrok, M., et al. "Treatment of hypertension with ascorbic acid." *Lancet.* 1999;354(9195):2048–49.

Chapter 6

Vickers, M.H., Ikenasio, B.A., Breier, B.H. "Adult growth hormone treatment reduces hypertension and obesity induced by an adverse prenatal environment." *J Endocrinol.* 2002 Dec;175(3):615–23.

Chen, J., He, J., Hamm, I., et al. "Serum antioxidant vitamins and blood pressure in the United States population." *Hypertension.* 2002 Dec;40(6): 810–6.

Abete, P., Testa, G., Ferrara, N., et al. "Cardioprotective effect of ischemic preconditioning is preserved in food-restricted senescent rats." *Am J Physiol Heart Circ Physiol.* 2002 Jun;282(6):H1978–87.

Steer, A.C., Carapetis, J.R., Nolan, T.M., et al. "Systematic review of rheumatic heart disease prevalence in children in developing countries: the role of environmental factors." *J Paediatr Child Health.* 2002 Jun;38(3):229–34.

Davidson, M.H., Maki, K.C., Karp, S.K., Ingram, K.A. "Management of hypercholesterolaemia in postmenopausal women." *Drugs Aging.* 2002; 19(3):169–78.

Mannion, J.D., et al. "Acute Electrical Stimulation Increases Extramyocardial Collateral Blood Flow After a Cardiomyoplasty." *Ann Thoracic Surg.* 56 (1993):1351–58.

Pickering, T.G., et al. "Tension and Hypertension." *JAMA.* Nov. 24, 1993, vol. 270, no. 20.

"Undo Pressure: Taking Control May Help Fight Hypertension." *Prevention.* Jan 1994:17–18.

Chapter 8

Mattioli, A.V., Bonetti, L., Zennaro, M., et al. "Prognostic value of iron, nutritional status indexes and acute phase protein in acute coronary syndromes." *Ital Heart J.* 2002 Mar;3(3):194–8.

Index

About the Authors

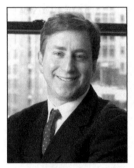 **Eric R. Braverman, M.D.**, is director of the Place for Achieving Total Health (PATH Medical) in New York City with satellite locations in Princeton, New Jersey and Penndel, Pennsylvania and director of the PATH Foundation, a nonprofit organization devoted to preventing and treating all aspects of brain chemical disorders as they relate to general health. He also served as director of research at the Robert C. Atkins Center for Alternative Therapies and chief clinical researcher at the Princeton Brain Bio Center.

In addition to his private practice and foundation work, Dr. Braverman frequently lectures at major medical conferences and has trained hundreds of physicians and health practitioners in his unique brain-based approach to health. He has appeared on numerous national radio and television programs from Larry King to the David Letterman Show and hosts a New York-based radio program called *Total Health*. He serves on the editorial boards of several scientific journals and is a frequent contributor to magazines such as *Let's Live, Total Health,* and *Harper's Bazaar.* He has written five books, among them *The Healing Nutrients Within* (Basic Health Publications, 2003) and *The Edge: The Path to Total Health and Longevity through the Balanced Brain* (Sterling Publishing, 2004), and is the author of more than 100 studies published in peer-reviewed medical research journals.

He is a diplomat of the American Board of Anti-Aging, with training at Harvard, Yale, and NYU medical schools, and is a recipient of the American Medical Association's Physician's Recognition Award.

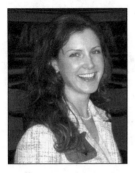

Dasha Braverman, B.S., R.P.A.-C., is founder and director of the Rainbow Wellness Center, a New York–based center that specializes in customizing nutrition plans for people suffering from chronic and lifestyle-related illnesses.

Mrs. Braverman is a graduate of Long Island University, where she received a Bachelor of Science degree and accreditation as a physician assistant. She began her early career teaching nutrition and wellness programs at various anti-aging clinics in the metropolitan area and, since then, has had the opportunity to work closely with some of the leading anti-aging experts and researchers, studying the impact of nutrition on health and well-being. She is a frequent guest lecturer at anti-aging seminars across the country.

Board-certified and licensed to practice nutrition in the state of New York, Mrs. Braverman is presently studying to receive a Masters of Science in preventive medicine. She is at work on a forthcoming book on the Rainbow Diet.